MECHANISM AND ROLE OF IMMUNOLOGICAL TOLERANCE

MONOGRAPHS IN ALLERGY

Vol. 3

Editors:

P. Kallós, Helsingborg
H. C. Goodman, Geneva
M. Hašek, Prague
T. Inderbitzin, Boston, Mass.

BASEL (Switzerland)   S. KARGER   NEW YORK

MECHANISM AND ROLE OF IMMUNOLOGICAL TOLERANCE

by T. HRABA, M.D.

Institute of Experimental Biology and Genetics,
Czechoslovak Academy of Sciences, Prague

19 68

BASEL (Switzerland)   S. KARGER   NEW YORK

MONOGRAPHS IN ALLERGY

S. Karger AG, Arnold-Böcklin-Strasse 25, CH-4000 Basel 11 (Switzerland)

CONTENTS

*"The scientist is the soldier of the truth.
This is correct even though the concept
of the truth changes and undergoes
evolution."*

LUDWIG HIRSZFELD

ACKNOWLEDGEMENTS

This monograph attempts to give a picture of the present state of knowledge of the problems implied in the title. I felt, however, that the picture would not be complete if it did not encompass the development of knowledge and of the hypotheses endeavouring to explain these phenomena and to incorporate them into more general concepts of the immunological process.

I trust I will be honorably excused for not considering the reason why the tremendous development which took place in the study of the suppression states of immunological reactions did not do so until the middle of this century. This is not only beyond my powers but would occupy far too much space. The methodical possibilities seemed to be available much earlier and, in fact, many suppression states were described before that time. I think that a clue to this rapid development is to be found in the discovery of transplantation tolerance. Its discovery stemmed from the important contribution to the problems of transplantation immunity provided by studies carried out by Sir PETER BRIAN MEDAWAR and his associates, starting in the 1940's.

An analysis of these relationships would be of much interest and value, and I hope it will be carried out. The purpose of this review of accomplishments and theories is different. I felt that familiarity with the development of the present concepts may ultimately help towards a better understanding of and a deeper insight into the present state of all the problems in this field.

In a monograph of this nature it would be impossible to consider all the aspects of this ever-increasing field of research, and therefore much will be left out that is well worth saying. The character of this Monograph Series permitted me to start from the results of Prof. HAŠEK and his group to which I have had the pleasure to belong since the very beginning of the investigations on tolerance. An attempt was made to deal with all the main problems in this field, but particular attention has been concentrated on the aspects related to the experiments carried out in the Institute of Experimental Biology and Genetics in Prague. This is also reflected in particular in the literature cited, as I did not try to give a complete review of the references to this subject. One of the reasons was that the authors of the first monograph published in this Series presented a very comprehensive list of publications relevant to immunological tolerance.

To Professor MILAN HAŠEK I owe many thanks for his kindness in reading the manuscript of this book and for his helpful suggestions, which have served to improve it. I am also most grateful to my colleagues of the Institute for their help at various stages of preparing the manuscript.

I. INTRODUCTION

The existence of immunological tolerance has been postulated by BURNET and FENNER [1949] to explain why the elimination of the body's own worn-out components does not lead to an immune reaction against them. The elimination of 'self' components is mediated by the same cells of the reticulo-endothelial system that eliminate foreign material against which an immune reaction takes place. Their hypothesis postulated that the immune reaction may take place only against those substances that are not recognized as 'self' by the organism. In their opinion the mechanism of self-recognition is not innate, genetically determined, but is acquired. They have assumed that at an early stage of development, when the ability for immune reactions has not yet developed, contact with antigenic substances does not pass without consequences for the reactivity of the organism and leads to the formation of a mechanism in the RES which is then able to differentiate 'self' from 'not-self'. Under normal conditions, the RES of the foetus meets only its own antigens because the maternal organism or the structure of the egg protects the developing organism from the invasion by microorganisms. The recognition mechanism is therefore limited to the organism's own substances. According to BURNET and FENNER there is no reason why any antigen encountered by the organism at this stage should not be recognized as 'self'. In formulating this hypothesis they started from the facts known at that time: erythrocyte chimaerism in twin cattle and TRAUB's observation of an asymptomatic type of infection by the virus of lymphocytic choriomeningitis.

In 1934, the colony of white mice in the Rockefeller Institute was found to be suffering from an infection caused by the virus of lymphocytic choriomeningitis [TRAUB, 1935]. The young animals were particularly affected, while the adults were immune against this disease. However, many adult animals appeared to carry and release the virus. In the following years, the disease increasingly acquired the nature of an asymptomatic infection [TRAUB, 1936a, 1936b, 1938,

1939]. After a short time a non-infected, virus-free colony was established from the original one. The rest of the infected colony was maintained and the infection retained its asymptomatic character. Mice in this colony were infected via intrauterine transmission of the virus, but the infection persisted practically throughout their life-span, and the lymphocytic choriomeningitis virus was present in undiminished concentrations in tissues of the infected animals. The injection of blood and of tissue suspensions from these mice into the brain of normal mice led to a disease similar to that observed at the beginning of the epidemic. The cause of the latent epidemic resided in the host, not in the changed character of the virus. The fact that latently infected mice were not capable of forming complement-fixing antibodies against the virus pointed to their altered immune reactivity.

This finding became the starting point for the experiments carried out by BURNET and his colleagues [BURNET et al., 1950] to provide an experimental verification of their hypothesis. Experiments were performed on chicken embryos which in comparison with mammalian embryos were more accessible to treatment. The antigens used for the induction of tolerance were a live influenza virus, bacteriophage or human erythrocytes. The expected result was, however, not obtained. After challenge antibody titres against these antigens were the same both in animals injected intraembryonally with the respective antigen and in control animals. Thus the first attempt to prove experimentally the hypothesis based on TRAUB's observation was not successful.

1. Natural Occurrence of Transplantation Tolerance

The tremendous development of cattle immunogenetics as a result of the preparation of a sufficient number of isoimmune monospecific antisera permitted a satisfactory antigenic differentiation of individual animals on the basis of their blood groups as early as in the first half of the 1940's. Although the majority of twin calves are dizygotic, their blood groups are generally identical. This contrasts with the situation in calves of the same parentage but born from different pregnancies. Such calves can be shown to differ in their blood groups. This discrepancy was explained by the finding of two erythrocyte populations in twin cattle by OWEN [1945].

The blood groups of cattle are mostly demonstrated by the haemolytic reaction. OWEN discovered the existence of erythrocyte chimaerism by observing that haemolysis by some reagents was not complete with erythrocytes of most cattle twins even though their blood groups were identical. This occurred in tests with antisera against the blood groups in which the twins differed. The antiserum then lysed only one of the two erythrocyte populations and the erythrocytes remaining intact after the reaction could not be lysed even when exposed again to the same antiserum. The cause of this chimaerism was seen by OWEN in an exchange of the haematopoietic precursor cells through anastomoses between the blood vessels of the foetal membranes of the twins. Such anastomoses were well known and were presumed to cause the occurrence of intersexuality, freemartinism, in the female member of twin pairs of unlike sex in cattle. OWEN assumed that cells from a twin partner settle in the other twin's tissues and produce their own type of erythrocytes. These erythrocytes are antigenically different from the host's erythrocytes. As a rule, erythrocyte chimaerism occurs in both twins, though the proportion of the two types of cell populations varies in each partner. As regards the qualitative antigenic composition, the mixed erythrocyte populations, as a whole, are alike in both such twins. This is conceivable, because two identical erythrocyte populations coexist in each of them.

BURNET and FENNER [1949] noticed the important aspect of this chimaerism. It is not surprising that the transplantation of haematopoietic cells may take place through a connection between the two circulations of the twins. The finding that this transplant may produce erythrocytes of its own antigenic type and thus different from the host's type is useful but also not surprising from the physiological point of view. BURNET and FENNER, however, directed attention to the fact that chimaerism may persist even in adult life, and this is surprising immunologically. In the early stages of individual development when the ability of embryos for immune reactions is not fully developed there is no danger for the transplant. However, immunologically mature recipients consistently destroy tissue homografts as a result of immune reaction towards them. This may be accounted for by a wide variability of individual antigens within an animal species so that practically no two individuals would possess an identical antigenic composition. An exception are monozygotic twins and members of inbred strains. Monozygotic twins actually represent a duplication of the same individual so that their genetically determined antigenic composition must be identical. In members of inbred strains complete genetic identity is achieved by inbreeding for many generations. In cattle twins erythrocyte chimaerism persists even after their immunological reactivity has matured. Their ability to react to haematopoietic tissues transplanted during their intrauterine life must have changed. Similarly, antigenically different erythrocytes produced by this transplant do not induce an immune reaction in their host although this happens almost invariably after their injection into other individuals.

Evidence on the suppression of transplantation immunity to individual antigens of a co-twin in cattle has been provided by MEDAWAR and his colleagues [ANDERSON et al., 1951; BILLINGHAM et al., 1952]. Monozygotic cattle twins are a valuable tool in genetic studies in this animal species, whose members are too expensive to be reared and mated in sufficient amounts merely for the observation of their inheritance, even though such studies ought to be carried out for practical purposes. The occurrence of genetically identical individuals – monozygotic twins – permits the accumulation of valuable information on the role of the genetic constitution and environment in their properties. The main difficulties encountered in using them for these purposes are a rare occurrence of monozygotic twin cattle and the determination of zygosity. Morphological diagnosis is not reliable. Determination by means of individual antigens appears to be the most accurate method so far. When MEDAWAR and his colleagues were carrying out their experiments, antisera for determining the blood groups were used in a few laboratories only. Therefore the high resolving power of the transplantation immune reaction seemed to be the simplest way. However, it appeared that skin grafts also survived in the majority of dizygotic twins, whereas skin grafts from siblings derived from different pregnancies, or from other closely related individuals, were rapidly rejected. This observation was an important contribution to the knowledge of the distribution of individual antigens in the tissues. Leucocytes were known to be capable of inducing transplantation immunity towards a skin graft from the same donor [MEDAWAR, 1946]. Such immunity could, however, be due to partial overlapping and not the identity of individual antigens on leucocytes and cells of the skin. The finding that haematopoietic cells induced tolerance both to themselves and to skin grafts pointed to the identity of their individual antigens responsible for transplantation immunity. If they shared only some of these antigens, then they might induce immunity in a foreign host on the basis of these common antigens, but tolerance elicited by one of these tissues would not be able to ensure tolerance to the other. The other tissue would possess the antigens that would be absent in the former tissue and would therefore not be tolerated. By means of transplantation tolerance it has since been shown that individual antigens responsible for transplantation immunity are probably identical in all tissues except for erythrocytes [HAŠEK et al., 1961].

The high incidence of erythrocyte chimaerism in cattle is due to the frequent occurrence of placental vascular anastomoses, which is the rule in twin cattle. In sheep, placental anastomoses and naturally induced tolerance are very rare. LAMPKIN [1953], using skin tests, did not find any tolerant animals in two pairs of sheep twins. His experiments, in spite of the small number of cases tested, indicated that the induction of transplantation tolerance in sheep twins would be rarer than in cattle twins, in which it would very probably have been found in at least one of the two pairs examined. The first case of erythrocyte chimaerism in sheep twins was described by STORMONT et al. [1953] in one of 26 pairs studied. In skin transplantation in nine pairs of sheep twins and one set of triplets we observed mutual tolerance to skin grafts in two individuals of opposite sex in the triplet litter [HRABA et al., 1956]. The grafts survived in good condition throughout the observation period, i.e. more than one year. The animals under study were given skin grafts from their litter-mates and from their mother. All these grafts, except for the tolerated one, were rejected. A similar situation was observed in the non-tolerant triplet. Rejection was complete within 18 days, except for the graft from the mother in one of the tolerant animals. This was still present on the 18th day, but only a scar was left of it by the 27th day. The prolongation in maternal graft survival might have been due to an antigenic overlap between mother and the tolerant sibling. The foetal membranes of animals from all these litters were examined. Vascular anastomoses between two placentae were found in the foetal membranes of triplets. MOORE and ROWSON (1958) observed tolerance to skin grafts in one of five pairs of sheep twins studied. This pair involved twins of opposite sex and the female twin was a freemartin. Later examination of their blood groups did not reveal erythrocyte chimaerism, but the blood groups of both animals were found to be identical [TUCKER, 1965]. SLEE [1963] also reported tolerance to skin grafts in three pairs of animals, two pairs of which came from a quadruplet litter and one pair from a triplet litter. Erythrocyte chimaerism was found in five animals out of these three pairs [TUCKER, 1965]. SLEE examined a total of 18 large litters

(3–5 lambs) and 7 twin litters. His findings and ours seem to suggest that tolerance occurs more frequently in sheep derived from large litters.

Placental vascular anastomoses are very rare in human dichorionic twins. On the other hand, they are frequent in human monochorionic twins, but insofar as hematopoietic cells pass and chimerism is established through them, it is impossible to prove this because, as a rule, monozygotic twins are involved. Nevertheless, a few cases of erythrocyte chimaerism have been reported in human dizygotic twins. The first case [DUNSFORD et al., 1953] was observed in a blood donor whose erythrocytes were strongly agglutinated by anti-A serum but large numbers – about 60% – of erythrocytes remained outside the agglutinates. The authors suspected that erythrocyte chimerism might have been involved. The blood donor was surprised when asked whether she had been born a twin. Her twin brother had died when three months old. The occurrence of erythrocyte chimerism as a result of somatic mutation was excluded because the two populations of erythrocytes differed in antigens controlled by three different loci. No signs of any effects of dispermy were obvious in the blood donor, nor did an analysis of the blood groups of the other living members of her family show any irregularities. The most feasible explanation was that in this case chimaerism resulted from the transplantation of hematopoietic cells of her brother. Her own erythrocytes were of the O group because she had O(H) substance and not A substance in her saliva. Thus the blood group of her twin could be found in her blood 25 years after his death. Later, another two cases of erythrocyte chimaerism were described in human twins [BOOTH et al., 1957; NICHOLAS et al., 1957], and here again O and A erythrocytes were mixed. In these cases, as in the previous one, the naturally occurring anti-A antibodies were suppressed. It is unlikely that their production would only be masked by foreign erythrocytes present in the circulation, since in these individuals neither increased haemolysis nor coating of erythrocytes with antibodies occurred.

Cellular chimaerism in human twins of unlike sex has also been demonstrated by means of sex-chromatin or sex chromosomes in the peripheral leucocytes [WOODRUFF and LENNOX, 1959; WOODRUFF et al., 1962]. However, in no case did the female member of any opposite-sex twin pair show signs of freemartinism.

In marmosets, unlike man, vascular anastomoses between the placentae of twins are extremely frequent. This is very surprising because a twin litter is the rule in them. The frequent occurrence of placental anastomoses between twin calves has been attributed to the fact that because of the rarity of multiple pregnancies no defence against their occurrence developed during the phylogenetic development; such a defence was supposed to exist in species in which larger litters are more frequent, e. g. in sheep. In marmosets, the female partner of heterosexual twins has never been a freemartin, in spite of a regular occurrence of vascular anastomoses. In three out of five male marmosets tested, BENIRSCHKE et al., [1962] found metaphases of opposite sex in the femoral bone marrow which was evidence of cell chimaerism established *in utero*.

In addition to the cases described, erythrocyte chimaerism has been reported in chickens born from double-yolked eggs [BILLINGHAM et al., 1956a] and in mink [RAPACZ et al., 1965], and it can be expected to occur with varying frequency in a number of other animal species.

2. Experimentally
Induced Transplantation Tolerance

Experimental studies based on the discovery of transplantation tolerance induced in dizygotic twins turned out to be very useful for the understanding of the phenomena of immunological tolerance.

MEDAWAR and his colleagues [BILLINGHAM et al., 1953] induced transplantation tolerance by injecting mouse embryos of the inbred CBA strain with suspensions of testicular, liver and spleen cells from A strain mice. The treated mice, when immunologically mature, were tested by skin grafts for their reactions to antigens of the donor strain. While the control animals of the CBA strain rejected allografts within 11 days, some of the treated animals tolerated them throughout the observation period, i. e., more than one year [BILLINGHAM et al., 1956a]. In some animals the rejection took place at the same time as in the controls, which was probably due to a technical error during injection of cells. Finally, in some cases, the survival of grafts was prolonged; even if this prolongation was considerable, the rejection did take place during the observation period. Similar results were obtained by these authors in White Leghorn chickens given intravenous injections of blood from Rhode Island Red embryonic donors on the 11th or 12th day of incubation. In five cases, the survival of skin grafts from blood donors was prolonged, and in two cases the grafts survived throughout the observation period (125 days). Much weaker tolerance to skin grafts performed later was obtained when the donor skin was transferred to the chorio-allantois of the recipients.

It appeared that immunological tolerance is not an 'all-or-nothing' phenomenon and that the survival of grafts may be prolonged for varying periods of time, even for the life-span of the recipients. Of importance for the elucidation of the mechanism of transplantation tolerance was the observation [BILLINGHAM *et al.*, 1956a] that tolerance of CBA mice to A grafts could be abolished by adoptive transfer of transplantation immunity [MITCHISON 1953, 1954]. The transfer of lymph node cells of CBA mice, in which transplantation immunity to cells of A strain individuals had been induced, into tolerant animals caused the rejection of the tolerated graft. It follows that tolerant animals lack immune lymphoid cells which might cause the rejection of the graft; if such a reaction may be brought about by transferred foreign cells, this is evidence of appropriate conditions for transplantation immune reaction against the tolerated graft to take place in the body of the tolerant animal. MEDAWAR and his associates, having been concerned for a long time with problems of transplantation immunity, were well aware of both the theoretical and the practical significance of this observation.

In the same year as MEDAWAR and his associates demonstrated experimentally that immunological tolerance can be produced, HAŠEK [1953 b] was successful in inducing it in a different model system. He developed the method of experimental embryonic parabiosis in avian embryos [HAŠEK, 1953 a] which was based on the fact that any tissue transplanted to the chorio-allantois of avian embryos becomes vascularized rapidly and richly. Since the immune mechanisms of the embryos are not yet mature, various allogeneic and xenogeneic grafts may survive on the chorio-allantoic membrane. The technique of embryonic parabiosis consists of exposing small parts of the chorio-allantois of two eggs and inserting a piece of tissue between the two bared chorio-allantoic membranes. The transplanted tissue is vascularized from the two chorio-allantoic membranes which become anastomosed. Through these connections an intensive exchange of blood between both partners takes place. In experimental embryonic parabiosis, as in natural parabiosis produced by vascular anastomoses between the foetal membranes of embryos from multiple pregnancies, the bodies of embryos are not joined. The parabiotic pairs separate spontaneously at the time of hatching: by closing the blood circulation in the foetal membranes the exchange of blood between the partners is discontinued and parabiosis disappears.

HAŠEK [1953 b] tested the change in immunological reactivity toward individual antigens of the partner by immunization with its erythrocytes. Chickens are known to have high immunological reactivity toward homologous erythrocyte antigens. Immunization of chickens with erythrocytes from any other one is almost always followed by the formation of immune isoagglutinins. If the immunization is sufficiently intensive, the antiserum reacts not only with the donor erythrocytes but also with those from all the other chickens with the exception of the antiserum producer [THOMSEN, 1934].

However, chicken parabionts did not produce any isoagglutinins when immunized with erythrocytes from their partners. After immunization with erythrocytes from other chickens they did produce isoagglutinins, but these also failed to react with their partners' erythrocytes [HAŠEK and HRABA, 1955 a]. Later on HAŠEK [1954] demonstrated that the parabionts also tolerated skin grafts from their partners.

Another advantage of experimental embryonic parabiosis as compared with the natural one is that embryos of diverse species can be joined [HAŠEK, 1953 a]. Such embryos well sustain the parabiotic union and hatch normally. The first combination of interspecific embryonic parabionts studied serologically was a combination of duck and chicken [FRENZL et al., 1955; HAŠEK and HRABA, 1955 a, b]. In both these species, natural heteroagglutinins against erythrocytes of the partner species are generally present. They could also be demonstrated in immunologically mature parabionts. The titre of immune heteroagglutinins against duck erythrocytes in chickens joined in parabiosis with ducks did not differ from that in control animals; on the other hand, ducks parabiosed with chickens showed lower titres of immune heteroagglutinins against chicken erythrocytes than the controls. A similar state of partial tolerance was obtained by SIMONSEN [1955] by injections of turkey blood into the chorio-allantoic vein of chicken embryos.

A higher degree of tolerance towards erythrocytes of the partner species was achieved in embryonic turkey-chicken parabionts [HAŠEK and HRABA, 1955 b; HRABA, 1956]. In one chicken parabiont turkey erythrocytes were detectable as long as 8 weeks after hatching. With regard to the life-span of turkey erythrocytes and the increase in the blood volume from the day of hatching, it was impossible that erythrocytes exchanged with the partner during parabiosis were involved.

Thus the cause must have been interspecific erythrocyte chimaerism established by foreign haematopoietic cells transferred during embryonic parabiosis [Hraba, 1956]. In later experiments, more cases of interspecific chimaerism were observed in the same combination of parabionts [Hašek et al., 1958, 1960]. The duration was generally limited (Table I), but in one turkey-chicken parabiont erythrocyte chimaerism persisted until the death of the bird at the age of more than one year [Hašek et al., 1959].

Table I. Persistence of partner's erythrocytes in turkey-chicken parabionts

Days after hatching	Number of chickens with persisting turkey erythrocytes	Number of turkeys with persisting chicken erythrocytes
<25	16	13
26–40	5	
41–80	5	
>81		1 (over one year)
Total	26	14

After Hašek et al. [1960].

Independently of these two groups of workers, S. H. Ripley, conducting experiments in the laboratory of R. D. Owen in 1953, was successful in inducing experimentally permanent erythrocyte chimaerism in rats by injections of foetal spleen and liver cells into the chorioallantoic vein [Owen, 1956].

When the first conference dealing with the subject was organized by the Royal Society three years after the first experimental results had been published, immunological tolerance was no longer a hypothetical phenomenon, but a phenomenon of which the main features were already known.

II. MECHANISM
OF IMMUNOLOGICAL TOLERANCE

1. The Concept
of Immunological Tolerance

The first definition of immunological tolerance was given by MEDA-
WAR and his colleagues [BILLINGHAM et al., 1956a]. It reads as follows:
'Tolerance represents the specific and systemic failure of the mechanism of immunological response which is brought about by exposing
embryos or very young animals to 'antigenic' stimuli, i. e. to stimuli
which would have caused older animals to have become sensitive or
immune. It is due to a primary central failure of the mechanism of the
immunological reaction, and not to some intercession, at a peripheral
level.' BILLINGHAM et al. assumed that this is a general immunologic
law and not only a phenomenon limited to transplantation immunity.
Later the term 'immunological tolerance' was used to name the
inhibition states induced by various antigens and presumed to be due
to the same mechanism as transplantation tolerance [CHASE 1959;
BUSSARD, 1963]. Although this aspect of tolerance as a general biological phenomenon was included in the above definition probably
on the basis of BURNET and FENNER's hypothesis [1949], it was
already at that time substantiated by a body of experimental data.
Of these, the most convincing appeared to be tolerance to heterologous serum proteins.

(a) Tolerance to Heterologous Serum Proteins

Almost at the same time as transplantation tolerance was induced experimentally, HANAN and OYAMA [1954] observed that repeated injections of bovine serum albumin (BSA), begun in the perinatal period,
led to complete suppression of antibody formation to this antigen in
rabbits. Similar results were obtained by DIXON and MAURER [1955]
with BSA and whole human serum, and by CINADER and DUBERT

[1955] with HSA. While HANAN and OYAMA [1954] and CINADER and DUBERT [1955] used relatively small amounts of antigen in one injection, DIXON and MAURER [1955] injected very large amounts: 500 mg BSA or 10 ml human serum/kg body weight (KBW) six times a week. The animals given such injections from the day of birth responded by non-immune elimination of antigen, not only after the cessation of serum injections but also after repeated challenge at least 11 months after the termination of the injection series. The same doses of antigen were used by DIXON and MAURER in adult rabbits. The immune reaction was again suppressed as shown by non-immune elimination of antigen, but mostly only over the period the antigen was present in the circulation after termination of the series of injections. When the antigen level decreased, accelerated elimination occurred in some cases showing the onset of an immune reaction. Normal immune reactivity appeared in all adult treated animals less than 6 months after cessation of the treatment. Adult animals had been injected with massive amounts of antigen for only 37 days and newborn animals for 98–112 days. The difference in reactivity observed might have been due, at least in part, to the longer time over which the antigen was injected and/or to the larger amount of antigen given. The experiments of JOHNSON *et al.* [1955] showed then that large amounts of BSA suppressed the immune response in at least some adult rabbits; suppression persisted even after the inducing dose of antigen had been eliminated, and lasted for at least 6 months.

A clear difference between very young and adult individuals emerged from experiments with newborn rabbits made tolerant by a single injection of antigen. SMITH and BRIDGES [1956] obtained such results using BSA. The smallest dose which completely suppressed antibody formation in all injected rabbits when immunized at the age of 4 months was 20 mg. DUBERT and PARAF [1957] observed that even a single injection of 1 mg HSA given at birth was capable of suppressing antibody formation completely. Similar doses elicit immune reactions in adult animals.

Tolerance to heterologous proteins has been induced in a variety of animal species. In most of them, it is, however, incomplete, or of shorter duration than in rabbits. In mice and chickens, experiments on the induction of tolerance were performed in both newborns and adults. In mice, the amount of antigen necessary to induce tolerance at birth is lower than that used in adult animals [DRESSER, 1961 b, 1962 a], while on the other hand, the difference between young and adult chickens is not pronounced: as a rule, a single injection of BSA given before or after hatching induces only partial and short-term tolerance [WOLFE et al., 1957; TEMPELIS et al., 1958 a, b]. Intraembryonic injection of HSA has similar effects [STEVENS et al., 1958]. We also observed a low degree of tolerance when we injected chickens with a single dose or repeated doses of HSA after hatching [IVÁNYI and HRABA, 1963]. A single injection of 2.5 g BSA/KBW which corresponded to the maximal dose used after hatching produced a stronger and more persistant tolerance in adult than in newly hatched chickens [MUELLER and WOLFE, 1961], though the inhibition did not seem to be complete [MUELLER, 1967]. Massive doses of HSA given in a single injection and especially in repeated injections led to the suppression of antibody formation in adult chickens which was comparable to that obtained through administration of antigen to very young animals [IVÁNYI et al., 1964 a].

It has been shown by DIXON and MAURER [1955] that tolerant animals formed antibody against antigenic impurities present in BSA preparations used for the induction of tolerance and for challenge. Their amount in these preparations was obviously too small to induce tolerance. A similar situation was observed by the same authors in experiments on induction of tolerance with whole human serum; they induced tolerance to its major but not its minor components. On the other hand, DOWNE [1955] did not find any precipitins against whole chicken serum after a course of injections commencing in the perinatal period. In experiments with human serum in which the same procedure of tolerance induction and immunization was used as in DOWNE's work, the treated animals produced precipitins detectable in reaction with whole human serum [HRABA, 1959]. The cause of the different results in DOWNE's experiments is not clear; our own findings were, however, repeatedly confirmed [HRABA and IVÁNYI, 1963; CINADER and DUBISKI, 1963]. The retained ability for immune reactions to antigenic impurities in protein preparations used for the induction of tolerance can thus serve as evidence for the specificity of immunological suppression in this phenomenon.

The central character of this suppression has been demonstrated both by antibody formation by lymphoid cells of nontolerant animals transferred to tolerant recipients [WEIGLE and DIXON, 1959; SMITH, 1960] and by inability of lymphoid cells of tolerant animals to form antibodies against the tolerated antigen after transfer to irradiated recipients [DIETRICH and WEIGLE, 1964].

(b) The Role of Age of the Recipient in Induction of Tolerance

Unresponsiveness to heterologous serum proteins met the criteria of immunological tolerance as stated in the given definition quoted above except for the point according to which tolerance is the state of unresponsiveness induced by the administration of antigen at an *early* age. If there is a difference in the inducibility of tolerance to these antigens between very young and adult animals, it may well be quantitative rather than qualitative. In immunologically mature animals, a skin homograft regularly represents an antigenic stimulus giving rise to transplantation immunity which then brings about destruction of the graft. On the other hand, in newborn chickens some skin homografts show a prolonged or permanent survival [CANNON and LONGMIRE, 1952; HRABA and HAŠEK, 1956]. Thus a skin graft alone can induce immunological tolerance in some newborn chickens. In newly-hatched ducks, the induction of tolerance by allogeneic skin grafts is the rule [HRABA and HAŠEK, 1956; HAŠEK, 1961]. Tolerance was induced in all five ducklings grafted even as late as 5 days after hatching, by the 7th day in two out of four, and by the 10th day in none of the ten ducklings tested [HAŠKOVÁ, 1957]. Tolerance could also be induced by skin grafts in newborn rabbits when the antigenic difference between donor and recipient was not too great [IVÁNYI and IVÁNYI, 1962; IVÁNYI, 1964].

However, convincing evidence of whether the recipient must be immunologically immature in order to be rendered tolerant was provided directly by the study of tolerance to allogeneic grafts. It appeared that transplantation tolerance could be induced even in adult mice [MARIANI et al., 1959; SHAPIRO et al., 1961; McKHANN, 1962; MARTINEZ et al., 1962, 1963]. Much larger amounts of cells are needed to induce tolerance in weanling and especially in adult mice in comparison with animals in the perinatal period. As viable cells are involved, these data are not accurate for an estimate of the exact amount of antigen required for the induction of tolerance. It is not known if and to what extent the injected cells multiply in the host body. An environment more favourable to the growth and multiplication of cells seems to be provided in newborn rather than in mature animals. Nevertheless, the difference in antigen requirements between newborn and older mice is considerable. The data of different authors vary as to the induction of transplantation tolerance in mature adults in case of a great antigenic difference between the donor and recipient [GOWLAND, 1965]. The possibility of inducing immunological tolerance in adult life, at least towards weak individual-specific antigens, shows that adult animals do not lack this ability.

Even if it were impossible to induce tolerance to strong individual antigens, the most likely explanation of this failure would be that it is not possible to inject the amount of antigen needed for the induction of tolerance. This appears to be the case, for example, with the suppression of immune reactions to heterologous erythrocytes in mice. Massive doses of erythrocytes capable of eliciting reduced antibody formation especially in primed animals are so large as to be hardly physiologically tolerable [ALBRIGHT and EVANS, 1965]. When, however, sheep erythrocytes were added to spleen cells in semipermeable chambers cultivated in the peritoneal cavity, a large dose of erythrocytes in relation to lymphoid cells could be used and strong suppression of antibody formation was achieved [ALBRIGHT and MAKINODAN, 1965; MAKINODAN et al., 1965].

The same seems to be true of transplantation tolerance, as is shown by the findings in animals with a chimaeric lymphoid system. Such chimaeras can be most easily produced experimentally when lymphoid cells are injected into very young or lethally irradiated recipients. Actually in this situation the reaction of transplanted immunologically competent cells to antigens of the recipients has been discovered. The possibility of this reaction has been suggested very early by SIMONSEN [1953]. In normally reactive hosts this phenomenon cannot be found because the transplanted cells are destroyed as a result of the hosts' immune reactions against them before the immune reaction against the host can occur. The graft versus host reaction by lymphoid cells used to induce tolerance in very young animals leads to runting of and general damage to the host. This pathological syndrome is designated as 'runt disease'. Lethally irradiated animals transplanted with haematopoietic tissue are protected against death at a time when unprotected animals die. This protection is, however, not permanent unless a syngeneic graft is used, or unless the host is compatible with the graft. This can happen when the host does not possess any antigen that is absent in the graft. In this situation the host is unable to induce an immune reaction in the graft. In other cases the animals protected with grafts frequently succumb, but their deaths occur later than in unprotected animals. This disease has been called the secondary disease, and, like runt disease, is due to graft-versus-host reaction [MICKLEM and LOUTIT, 1966]. In both cases the immunological reactivity of the host is absent or depressed, in the first case by tolerance induced by the graft, and in the second by X-irradiation. The graft surviving under these conditions may therefore display an immune reaction against the host.

It is not surprising that transferred lymphoid cells can elicit an immune reaction in their new host. Earlier experiments have already shown that lymphoid cells transfer delayed hypersensitivity (CHASE, 1945] or antibody production [HARRIS et al., 1952, 1954; ŠTERZL, 1955] to other animals. However, in the case of an immune reaction of the graft against the host the graft reacts against antigens of the organism in which it produces the immune reaction. Thus the cell autonomy of the immune reaction has clearly been proved. The secondary disease and the resultant mortality were eliminated or substantially reduced when embryonic haematopoietic cells were used as protective grafts [LENGEROVÁ, 1958, 1959; BARNES et al., 1958; FELDMAN and YAFFE, 1958; ILBERY et al., 1958; UPHOFF, 1958b].

A young graft could evidently acquire tolerance to the antigens of its host and thus the immune reaction against the host was prevented. That this hypothesis is true has been confirmed by experiments on transplantation of lethally irradiated recipients with haematopoietic cells from donors of two different inbred strains. Insofar as both donors were embryos, reciprocal tolerance could be induced (LENGEROVÁ et al., 1961; LENGEROVÁ and MICKLEM, 1962; LENGEROVÁ, 1962, 1963]. In non-inbred irradiated recipients it has even been possible to induce polyvalent transplantation tolerance to skin grafts from any donor when protected by a pool of cells from a sufficient number of embryonic donors after lethal irradiation [LENGEROVÁ, 1960]. The cause of this polyvalent tolerance is that the antigens of cells from individual donors induce tolerance in cells of all the other donors. The individual antigenic specificity is due to a relatively small number of antigens being present irregularly in animals of the same species. In each of them a unique mosaicism of these antigens occurs. The number of the possible combinations even of a few antigens is so great that it is very unlikely that two individuals will ever possess an identical antigenic mosaic. On the other hand, a group consisting of a relatively small number of individuals will most probably possess all individual antigens of the given population. If the injected embryonic cells derived from a sufficient number of donors acquire tolerance to antigens of all cells in the inoculum, it is unlikely that any individual in the given population would contain antigens other than those present in the pooled inoculum and of which this chimaeric recipient would not be tolerant.

If a pool of adult and embryonic cells was used for the inoculation of lethally irradiated recipients, then adult cells predominated and the embryonic graft was eliminated evidently as a result of an immune graft to graft reaction [LENGEROVÁ et al., 1961; CLARKE et al., 1962]. Even in this experimental arrangement it has been possible to suppress the elimination of embryonic grafts, obviously as a result of tolerance induction in cells of adult grafts [LENGEROVÁ and POLÁČKOVÁ, 1963]. It was, however, not sufficient to adjust the proportion of embryonic and adult cells in favour of the embryonic ones during their inoculation after irradiation. Embryonic cells had to be injected repeatedly. Evidently the amount of antigen required for the induction of tolerance in adult cells was very high.

The view that tolerance to very strong individual antigens can be induced even in adult animals, but using extremely high doses of antigen, has been supported by the finding that the graft cells do not react against the host's antigens in radiation chimaeras surviving secondary disease [COLE and DAVIS, 1961; PREHN and THURSH, 1962; VAN BEKKUM, 1962, 1963]. Long-term co-existence with the host's antigens showed the same effect on adult spleen cells which had been injected to elicit tolerance in newborn mice and which at first had reacted against their host [MICHIE et al., 1961]. The excess of the host's antigens is apparently sufficient to induce tolerance in these cases.

It is important that transplantation tolerance induced in young adults has been shown not to differ from that induced neonatally: in both cases, specific suppression of immune reaction is involved. The tolerant animals are cell chimaeras and the unresponsiveness is brought about by central failure of the mechanism of immunological reaction demonstrable by the adoptive transfer [GOWLAND, 1965]. Evidence is lacking for transplantation tolerance induced in mature adults, but there is no indication that the situation might be different in them.

It has also been possible to induce tolerance to allogeneic erythrocytes in adult ducks by means of exsanguination transfusion [HAŠEK and PUZA, 1962a, b]. The donor erythrocytes persisted in tolerant animals as long as the autologous ones, i.e., for 25–35 days, while in control animals allogeneic erythrocytes were eliminated within 10 days. Tolerance to skin grafts was, however, not induced by this treatment, although it was easily elicited during embryonic parabiosis. An exact comparison of the quantitative relationships in young and adult animals is not easy here, but the 'inducibility' of tolerance is obviously much more difficult in adults. An attempt to induce tolerance by exsanguino-transfusion in adult animals between two closely related species of ducks – the domestic and the muscovy duck – was not successful. Failure was probably due to the great antigenic difference.

An important contribution to the question of whether the difference in 'inducibility' of transplantation tolerance between newborn and adult animals is qualitative or merely quantitative has been the discovery that young animals are capable of an immune response to antigens of allogeneic cells even in the perinatal period. The possibility of inducing transplantation immunity in newborn mice by the use of lower doses of cells than those eliciting tolerance has been pointed out by HOWARD and MICHIE [1962]; BRENT and GOWLAND [1962a, 1963]. In chickens which can still be rendered tolerant by injection of allogeneic cells given after hatching, the chick embryos have already proved to be capable of inhibiting the graft-*versus*-host reaction elicited by injection of allogeneic cells [ISACSON, 1959; SOLOMON and TUCKER, 1963]. This inhibition seems to be due to an immune reaction of the embryo against the graft. The sensitization of chicken embryos may even lead to an accelerated rejection of skin grafts shortly after hatching [SOLOMON, 1963].

There is nothing surprising in the finding that transplantation immunity is observed at such early stages of individual development, since it may commence still earlier in other animal species. For example, sheep embryos are able to reject allogeneic skin grafts during the second trimester of gestation [SCHINKEL and FERGUSON, 1953], and a similar situation seems to exist in rabbits [BILLINGHAM et al., 1956a; PORTER, 1960]. However, it is important that the ability to develop transplantation immunity appears in mice and chickens at a time when tolerance is easy to induce by relatively small amounts of allogeneic cells. These amounts are small, at least in comparison with those needed to induce tolerance in animals only several days older.

The evidence presented suggests that there are only quantitative differences in inducibility of tolerance between very young and adult individuals.

(c) Effects of Irradiation
and Immunosuppressive Drugs on Induction of Tolerance

DIXON and MAURER [1955] found that massive doses of HSA led either to a delay in antibody formation or to its short-term suppression in adult rabbits. If, however, the animals were exposed to a non-lethal X-ray dose (400 r) before a series of injections started, much greater suppression of antibody formation was achieved. Three months later, none of these animals showed an immune elimination of antigen injected, and no immune elimination was apparent over the whole observation period, i.e., 6 and 9 months. Previous irradiation thus increased the effect of the tolerance-inducing dose.

The observation that irradiation facilitates the induction of tolerance to heterologous proteins has been confirmed and further analysed by NACHTIGAL and FELDMAN [1963]. Otherwise immunogenic doses of HSA or BSA given to rabbits irradiated with 550 r were shown to suppress the formation of antibodies against these antigens on subsequent challenge. The degree of this suppression decreased as the interval between irradiation and antigen injection that ought to induce unresponsiveness was prolonged.

SCHWARTZ and DAMESHEK [1959] started together with the injection of BSA in adult rabbits, a two-week course of 6-MP administration. The antigen injected did not elicit an immune reaction. On an additional injection of BSA several weeks later, the treated animals eliminated the injected antigen in a non-immune fashion. Thus, using this drug, tolerance has been induced in this experiment with a dose of antigen that elicits immunity in normal animals. GOH et al. [1961], conducting similar experiments, concluded that they could not induce tolerance to BGG under these conditions. It seems, however, likely that the absence of the immune phase of antigen elimination in two out of six of their experimental rabbits during challenge performed a month later is a manifestation of induced tolerance. Some differences in genetic and breeding conditions might have played a part and caused a considerably higher mortality of the animals used in the experiments of GOH et al. compared to those of SCHWARTZ and DAMESHEK. Besides this, the small dose of antigen (20 mg BGG/KBW) might be the cause of the failure in the experiments of GOH et al. In their later experiments SCHWARTZ and DAMESHEK [1963] pointed to the importance of antigen dose for drug-induced tolerance. With BSA, the lowest dose regularly eliciting tolerance was 66 mg/KBW. The possibility of inducing tolerance to BSA and HSA by means of 6-MP has also been confirmed by other authors [FELDMAN et al., 1962; NACHTIGAL and FELDMAN, 1963].

In guinea-pigs, tolerance to heterologous proteins by means of 6-MP could not be induced [HUMPHREY, 1963], but success was recorded when cyclophosphamide was used [Maguire and Maibach, 1961; Salvin and Smith, 1964].

As regards transplantation immunity, it has been found by a number of authors on various models of both the host-*versus*-graft and graft-*versus*-host reaction that some immunosuppressive drugs facilitate the induction of transplantation tolerance in young and mature adults [Uphoff, 1958a; McLaren, 1961; Uphoff and Pitkin, 1962; Russell, 1962; Woodruff, 1962; Medawar, 1963; Skowron-Cendrzak, 1964; Hilgert, 1965]. The convenience of various drugs depends on different factors such as the animal species, the nature and form of antigen injected, etc. The right temporal relation between injection of antigen and of drug is of equal importance as in the case of tolerance induction by means of irradiation. In view of the practical importance of this method of tolerance induction, many experiments dealt with the screening of suitable drugs and the determining of the best way of using them for this purpose. The drugs, which were shown to have this capacity, were some antimetabolites and alkylating agents while other immunosuppressive drugs were supposed to be ineffective [Humphrey, 1962]. I would like to report on some experiments in which this effect has been achieved by one of these drugs, namely cortisone. Devenyi *et al.* [1957a, 1957b, 1958a, 1958b, 1962] found that allogeneic grafts of thyroid and parathyroid in rats were rejected within 30 days. The treated recipients, partly thyroidectomized, partly with their own intact thyroid, were given 15 mg cortisone in 6 doses within 11 days of transplantation. The animals were then successively sacrificed, and the grafts were histologically examined. Most of the grafts appeared to be in good condition throughout the observation period of 300 days for thyroidectomized animals and 230 days for non-thyroidectomized ones. The reduction in the dose of cortisone by shortening the injection series resulted in an impaired survival of the grafts [Devényi *et al.*, 1958c]. Using ^{131}I, 23 of 28 grafts analysed on the 106th, 170th and 227th day after transplantation were shown to be capable of taking up iodine; this indicated that their parenchyma survived and was capable of specific functions [Devenyi *et al.*, 1958d]. Similar results showing a permanent effect of cortisone on skin graft survival in chickens were obtained by Cannon and Longmire [1952]. On the other hand, Meyer *et al.* [1964] did not observe any effect of corticosterone in this respect; when they interrupted the drug supply, the rejection of grafts was accelerated. It is likely that allogeneic thyroid grafts are less sensitive to transplantation immunity and that, for this reason, they were more suitable for detecting tolerance following cortisone treatment.

Sublethal doses of irradiation are also effective in facilitating the induction of transplantation tolerance in adult animals [MICHIE and WOODRUFF, 1962; MEDAWAR, 1963; FEFER and DAVIES, 1963]. RYCH-LÍKOVÁ and CHUTNÁ [1965] were successful in obtaining polyvalent tolerance in irradiated random-bred adult mice using a pool of embryonic cells from various donors. The injection of a cell mixture alone induced polyvalent tolerance in newborn mice similar to that obtained in ducks [HAŠEK and HAŠKOVÁ, 1958; HAŠEK, 1959] and rats [BILLINGHAM and SILVERS, 1959; KOLDOVSKÝ, 1961a, b]. This could not be achieved in adult mice without irradiation, even if the largest possible doses of pooled cells were used.

Data available at present show that non-specific reduction of immunological reactivity by chemical or physical agents generally results in an enhanced inducibility of tolerance, due to quantitative rather than qualitative changes in the respective apparatus. This can be inferred from the fact that the irradiation doses that may facilitate the induction of tolerance do not completely suppress antibody formation. In this connection, the results of NATHAN et al. [1961] are of interest. Agglutinin formation elicited by the injection of a 0.25 ml 30% sheep erythrocyte suspension was only slightly less in mice treated with 6-MP than in the controls. However, when the dose of sheep erythrocytes was increased three times, agglutinin formation was completely suppressed in the treated animals.

These findings therefore also lend support to the view that the causes underlying the differences in inducibility of tolerance in very young and adult animals are quantitative and not qualitative.

(d) Immunological Paralysis

As the induction of unresponsiveness in the intraembryonic stage or in very young animals is not a necessary characteristic of immunological tolerance, there is no difficulty in including immunological paralysis in the group of tolerance phenomena. Immunological paralysis has been discovered earlier than transplantation tolerance. Since it has been induced in adult animals, its inclusion among the phenomena of immunological tolerance has been accepted with some reservation.

Immunological paralysis is a state of inhibition that may be induced in mice by injecting them with a relatively small amount of bacterial polysaccharides. In most cases, pneumococcal polysaccharides were used and injected in a single dose or repeatedly (Felton and Ottinger, 1942; Felton, 1949; Felton et al., 1955a). Pneumococcal polysaccharide is a complete antigen for mice, and relatively small amounts are capable of eliciting immunity that can easily be tested by resistance against infection by viable pneumococci. Antibody formation can be suppressed by doses approximately 10–100 times higher than the optimal immunizing dose. Animals paralysed by a sufficient dose of polysaccharide lose their ability to develop immunity against the strain of pneumococci from which the polysaccharide has been prepared. The ability for immune reactions to polysaccharides of other pneumococcal strains is, however, retained in paralysed animals. Thus the suppression achieved is specific.

The polysaccharide injected during the induction of immunological paralysis persists for a long time in the body. Its presence could be demonstrated by showing that extracts from tissues of paralysed mice were capable of eliciting immunity in other mice against the polysaccharide used for the induction of paralysis in the donor [Felton et al., 1955b]. The polysaccharide could be demonstrated in paralysed mice even after more than one year, although its concentration measured in this way seemed to decrease considerably with time (Felton et al., 1955b; Stark, 1955]. In comparison with this reduction in antigenicity, the amount of ^{14}C isotopes employed for labelling polysaccharide to be used in induction of immunological paralysis, remains unchanged in tissues of paralysed mice throughout the observation period. Thus the question remains open whether or not the degraded material, in spite of losing its antigenicity, fulfils some function in maintaining tolerance.

The antigen persisting in tissues of paralysed mice is also capable of binding passively introduced antibodies. In passive protection of paralysed mice against infection, two to four times more antibody had to be used than in untreated mice [Felton et al., 1955a]. The rapid elimination of passively administered rabbit antibodies against pneumococcal polysaccharide in paralysed mice as compared with normal mice [Dixon et al., 1955] is, to a large extent, due to immune reactions of the mouse recipients to rabbit γ-globulin [Gitlin et al., 1961]. Rabbit antibody bound to polysaccharide in vivo or in vitro accelerates antibody formation against rabbit γ-globulin in mice. However, the binding of passively introduced antibodies in paralysed mice really does exist, as has been shown by means of mouse antibodies. By neutralization of passively administered mouse antibodies against poly-saccharide used for the induction of paralysis in the recipients of serum it has been possible to determine the half-life of polysaccharide in the body [SISKIND and PATERSON, 1964]. The half-life was 5 days during the first 10 days after injection of antigen; then it was markedly prolonged, becoming 50 days between 11 and 70 days. The reason for this change is not known. It is not caused by an immune reaction of the host against the given antigen. The half-life of polysaccharide is the same, regardless of the amount given. If the shorter half-life after the injection were due to antibody formation, the half-life of smaller doses of antigen would be shorter than that of the larger doses.

The presence of antigen in the paralysed organism and the binding of passively administered antibodies by this antigen has led to the view that immunological paralysis is in fact no suppression of anti-body formation. A hypothesis has been formulated [KAPLAN et al., 1950; STARK, 1955] that paralysed mice do form antibodies, but these, as the passively administered ones, are bound by antigen present in the body and the resultant state simulates the suppression of immune reactions. Quantitative studies of the amount of antigen present in tissues after the paralysing injection [SISKIND and PATERSON, 1964], however, show that this amount is less than that needed for binding antibodies formed by normal mice in response to the immunizing dose of polysaccharide. Further evidence of immunological paralysis being due to the suppression of antibody formation may be seen in the abo-lition of paralysis by the adoptive transfer of immunity [NEEPER and SEESTONE, 1963; BROOKE and KARNOFSKY, 1961]. In full agreement with these findings are the observations that the lymphoid cells of paralysed animals transferred adoptively to normal recipients fail to produce antibodies even in this environment without antigen excess.

It follows from the above statements that immunological paralysis fulfils all the requirements necessary for it to be regarded as a state of immunological tolerance. In recent years the possibility of its induc-tion in newborn mice has also been studied. With type II pneumo-coccal polysaccharide, it has been shown that a similar dose induces paralysis in newborn mice and in young adults [SISKIND et al., 1963]. Of importance was the finding that immunity could be elicited in newborn mice by smaller doses of polysaccharide than those used to induce paralysis. With type I pneumococcal polysaccharide [NEEPER, 1964], 14-day-old mice were found to be more susceptible to the in-duction of paralysis than newborn or adult mice. Finally, with type III pneumococcal polysaccharide, the amount of antigen needed to induce paralysis was 5–20 times higher in mice 25–66 weeks old than in young ones (6–11 weeks of age) [BROOKE, 1965b]. No difference in the required dose was noted between newborn and young animals when inducing immunological paralysis with this type of polysaccharide. Thus immunological paralysis can be induced in newborn mice, but this age category does not seem to be more appropriate than young adults. This may be due to the fact that the ability of newborn mice for immune reactions towards these antigens is already sufficiently mature.

(e) Tolerance to Viral and Bacterial Antigens

Attempts to induce immunological tolerance by injections of viral and bacterial antigens into embryos or newborn animals were not successful [BURNET et al., 1950; COHN, 1957; SMITH and BRIDGES, 1958; GOWLAND and OAKLEY, 1960; FESTENSTEIN and BOKKENHEU-SER, 1961], or led only to a reduction in antibody formation in treated animals upon challenge [BUXTON, 1954; KERR and ROBERTSON, 1954; ŠTERZL and TRNKA, 1957; FRIEDMAN and GABY, 1960; WICHER and ROGALOWA, 1960; GOŚCICKA, 1963; NAGY, 1963]. The situation was very similar to that encountered in experiments on the induction of tolerance to heterologous cells [BURNET et al., 1950; SIMONSEN, 1955; HAŠEK and HRABA, 1955a], where the tolerance, if demonstrable at all, was as a rule only partial. In complete contrast to these results were the findings relative to the induction of transplantation tolerance to homologous cells [BILLINGHAM et al., 1953; HAŠEK, 1954]. These findings raised the question of whether it would ever be possible to induce complete tolerance to antigens of phylogenetically distant sources [HAŠEK and HRABA, 1955b; NOSSAL and MÄKELÄ, 1961]. An exception was tolerance to heterologous serum proteins. The fact that it is not caused by some specific property of these substances was proved by CINADER et al. [1958], who were successful in inducing tolerance to bovine ribonuclease in rabbits. Strong tolerance was, however, obtained also to cells of individuals belonging to some closely related species [HRABA, 1956; HAŠEK et al., 1960]. Thus the possibility remained that protein antigens were not sufficiently distant substances.

An answer to this question has been given by the results obtained in experimental models permitting the detection of immunological response to a single antigenic substance of a distant phylogenetic provenience. Immunological paralysis to bacterial polysaccharides could not well serve as an argument, as in the 1950's its mechanism was still not clear and it had been induced in adult animals.

The first experiment in which strong tolerance to a substance derived from a phylogenetically distant organism had been achieved was the induction of tolerance to yeast glucoso-6-phosphate-dehydrogenase (GPDH) in newborn rabbits [BUSSARD, 1957, 1960]. Newborn rabbits were injected daily with 0.2 mg protein preparation from the day of birth up to 10 days. Challenge was performed in the 7th month and the antibodies formed were detected by inhibition of enzymatic activity of GPDH. Neutralizing antibodies were not demonstrable in the majority of the treated animals, and in animals that had formed them the titres were lower than in the controls. The degree of tolerance obtained was high, although non-precipitating and non-neutralizing antibodies were present in serum of most of the tolerant animals; these antibodies were demonstrable by precipitation of complexes they formed with GPDH at a 35% concentration of ammonium sulphate.

NOSSAL et al. [1965] were successful in inducing tolerance to Salmonella adelaide flagellin in newborn rats. They prepared a highly purified preparation of this protein, which is a strong antigen for rats [ADA et al., 1965a]. It has been possible to induce complete suppression of the formation of serologically detectable antibodies by a course of injections of small doses of flagellin starting on the day of birth, or by a single injection of a larger amount of this substance into newborn animals. It is, however, likely that this tolerance is not complete. This possibility seems to be suggested by the immune localization of antigen in the lymph nodes of tolerant animals which is probably due to opsonizing antibodies [NOSSAL and ADA, 1964]. Nevertheless, the suppression of the immune reaction is very strong here because, as stated above, flagellin is a strong antigen capable of eliciting very intensive immune reactions in rats.

Attempts to induce tolerance to influenza virus in chickens [BURNET et al., 1950] and mice [NOSSAL, 1957] failed and contrasted with TRAUB's observation of asymptomatic infection with lymphocytic choriomeningitis virus (LCM) in mice infected in utero [TRAUB, 1939]. A mild course of the infection with this virus in newborn mice has been confirmed [WHITNEY, 1951; HOTCHIN, 1958], but the main evidence of its being due to the recipient's tolerance has been provided by TRAUB's observation that these mice fail to form complement-fixing antibodies against LCM virus. This finding has been confirmed by other authors [WEIGAND and HOTCHIN, 1961; VOLKERT *et al.,* 1964], but the evidence is too weak to draw such a conclusion. The finding that the state of viraemia in these animals can be abolished by an adoptive transfer of lymphoid cells from immune or even normal individuals [VOLKERT and LARSEN, 1964, 1965a, 1965b], however, offers strong support to this view.

The infection with LCM virus itself does not seem to be dangerous for mice. This conclusion is supported by the finding that tissue cultures infected with this virus do not show any signs of damage. The clinical symptoms may be due to an immune reaction induced by the virus in the host. If the host is not capable of this reaction, the infection is not accompanied by any signs of the disease. This has been observed in young animals, but irradiation or antimetabolites given to adult mice simultaneously with the virus inoculum were also shown to lead to asymptomatic infection [ROWE, 1956; HAAS and STEWART, 1956; HOTCHIN and WEIGAND, 1961b; COLINS *et al.*, 1961]. It is likely that such treatment may facilitate the induction of tolerance to the virus in adult mice.

In adoptive transfer of immunity to mice with an asymptomatic infection with LCM virus no clinical signs of the disease were apparent during the elimination of the virus from the body. Thus they seem to be due only to some type of immune reaction to the virus. This seems to be a delayed-type hypersensitivity reaction.

If the pathogenic agent were itself capable of damaging the organism, then the occurrence of tolerance to it would impair the survival of the infected individual. An example of this is immunological paralysis to pneumococcal polysaccharides, which prevents the organism from acquiring immunity to infection with this microorganism. The infectious agents are, however, complex, possessing a number of antigenic substances. These can induce various kinds of immune reactions; some of these reactions are very effective in the defence against infection, although some may be harmful to the organism. As a rule, an evaluation of this situation is not easy and it is even more difficult to estimate the changes occurring in the course of infection when the immune reaction has been influenced in some way. For example, MIL-GROM *et al.* [1958] injected live BCG into guinea-pig embryos. Because of the low level of oxygen in the embryo the environment is not favourable to the growth of the inoculum, which is destroyed. The treated guinea-pigs together with control animals were infected with *Mycobacterium tuberculosis* when immunologically mature. The course of infection was milder in the treated animals and they also survived longer than the controls. Tuberculin hypersensitivity was absent in the treated animals before challenge, so interaembryonal injection did not seem to induce immunity. The authors have interpreted this finding by assuming that the milder course of infection was due to the fact that the intraembryonic administration of BCG had induced tolerance which then led to a diminished intensity of the immune reaction to *Mycobacterium tuberculosis*. They assumed that at least some allergic reactions elicited by these bacteria damaged the organism, and that their suppression was beneficial. This interpretation is subject to some doubt, according to the results of WEISS and WELLS [1957]; WEISS [1958]. These authors injected guinea-pig embryos with old tuberculin or live or killed BCG. Old tuberculin did not induce sensitivity and after subsequent immunization reduced the capacity for sensitization. Killed and live BCG led directly to sensitization in many animals inoculated *in utero*. Animals injected with killed vaccine and not developing hypersensitivity had a reduced ability to form it upon later immunization. On the other hand, animals inoculated with live BCG, in which hypersensitivity did not develop, were hypersensitive after a new immunization as rapidly as control animals. The question of whether the suppression of reactivity observed in these experiments after an intrauterine injection of old tuberculin and killed BCG is immunological tolerance or immune deviation will not be considered here. A regular occurrence of hypersensitivity after the injection of live BCG, however, seems to suggest that the prolonged survival of animals inoculated *in utero* with live BCG, observed by MILGROM and his associates, might have been a manifestation of immunity induced by the intrauterine injection. This seems to be supported by the findings of REES and GARBUTT [1961], in whose experiments mice given an intrauterine injection of live BCG or of killed virulent strain of *M. tuberculosis* survived longer after infection at the age of 5–6 weeks. In their tissues, however, less bacilli were found than in control animals. The authors see in these results evidence that the prolonged survival of treated mice was due to immunity rather than to tolerance. Moreover, their mice injected *in utero* showed, at the age of 5–6 weeks, without any further treatment, signs of delayed hypersensitivity to tubercle bacilli which was evidently the result of immunity caused by infection *in utero*.

Recently, tolerance to pathogenic agents has been most widely studied on oncogenic viruses where it appeared to play a very significant role. Since this aspect of the subject is not directly related to the question of the mechanism of immunological tolerance, it will not be considered here, but references to it can be found in Svoboda's review [1966]. In this connection it is worth recalling that Traub [1941] observed an increased incidence of lymphomatosis in mice with asymptomatic infection with LCM virus.

Although the phylogenetic distance of the source of antigen does not obviously impede the induction of complete tolerance, the possibility remains that this factor may play a role in the ease with which tolerance can be induced. To study this reationship a substance of the same chemical nature but of different provenience must be used, as the chemical nature of antigen has been shown to be of decisive importance in tolerance induction. For such comparisons HSA and duck serum albumin were used in our experiments. Complete tolerance was induced in newborn rabbits, but no difference was found as to its inducibility by these two antigens [Hraba and Iványi, 1963]. On the other hand, it has been shown by Iványi and Valentová [1966] that in chickens tolerance to duck albumin could be induced with a lower dose and persisted longer than tolerance to HSA. The results seem to be in agreement with findings in mice [Dietrich, 1963; Dietrich and Weigle, 1963]. Although with mammalian serum proteins of various species it was impossible to demonstrate a relationship between inducibility and degree of tolerance on the one hand and their antigenicity and rate of catabolism on the other; the corresponding avian serum proteins were inferior in this respect. Thus, this relationship may play a certain role, but not as significant one as was presumed.

(f) The Role of Antigen in Maintaining Tolerance

An important contribution to understanding the nature of immunological tolerance has been provided by Smith and Bridges [1958], who induced tolerance by a single injection of various amounts of BSA in newborn rabbits. This appeared to be a transient state; its duration lengthened as the amount of injected antigen increased. In most of the rabbits, tolerance began to disappear after injection of 100 mg between 135 and 189 days, after 10 mg between 90–135 days and after 1 mg between 70–90 days [Smith, 1961]. This finding differed from the results of Dixon and Maurer [1955] and of Cinader and Dubert [1955, 1956] since in their experiments tolerance to heterologous serum proteins seemed to be permanent. The permanence of tolerance in these experiments was found to depend on testing the animals with repeated injections of the tolerated antigen. SMITH and BRIDGES [1958] reported that even very small amounts of antigen could maintain tolerance if given to tolerant animals before the tolerant state disappeared. It was then postulated that tolerance can be maintained practically permanently by repeated injections of relatively small amounts of antigen.

This relation between duration of tolerance and persistence of antigen which had induced it could not be easily detected in tissue transplantation experiments. In the very beginning, such tolerance could be induced only by living cells. The induced transplantation tolerance then resulted in the establishment of a cell chimaera, as the immune reaction eliminating the inoculated cells under normal conditions was suppressed. Cells of the inoculum might then become a permanent source of antigen for maintaining tolerance.

It might be expected that the question as to whether cell chimaerism will always be a prerequisite for maintaining tolerance might be decided by elucidating the situation with split-tolerance to cell antigens. In such cases some antigens of cells that have induced tolerance are tolerated while others are not. Since in these cases the host reacts to non-tolerated antigens carried by the same cell as tolerated antigens the chimaera should be eliminated. However, in experiments of BRENT and COURTENAY [1962] both tolerated and non-tolerated antigens were shown to persist in the spleen of split-tolerant animals, and thus the chimaera did not disappear though the recipient reacted against the donor cells in an immune fashion. Thus the situation with partial tolerance did not refute the hypothesis that cellular chimaerism was responsible for maintaining transplantation tolerance. The role of cellular chimaerism in maintaining tolerance was clearly demonstrated in experiments of HAŠEK [1963a] on embryonic parabionts between Peking ducks and muscovy ducks. In this interspecific combination, erythrocyte chimaerism frequently occurs. It was observed that its disappearance was associated with loss of tolerance to erythrocytes. It is possible that in these parabionts erythrocyte chimaerism disappears for non-immune reasons, as the skin grafts from a donor of the partner species can be further tolerated. This conclusion is not unequivocal because the onset of immunity to erythrocytes during persisting tolerance to skin grafts or *vice versa* has been observed in both intraspecific [ŠTARK *et al.*, 1960, 1961a, 1961b, 1961c, 1962; HAŠEK *et al.*, 1961] and interspecific relationships [HAŠEK and HORT, 1960]. The interspecific chimaerism in parabionts between muscovy and Peking duck may be abolished by the passive transfer of antiserum against cells of the graft. In this case, tolerance to erythrocytes also disappears, as in spontaneous disappearance of chimaerism. This can be prevented by injecting animals, in which chimaerism had been abolished in this way, twice weekly with erythrocytes in amounts capable of eliciting immune reactions in normal animals. By removing the source of tolerated antigen in the body tolerance is lost; in contrast, tolerance can be maintained by supplying antigen from without after its source in the body has been removed.

On the other hand, in long-lasting radiation chimaeras it has been shown that after back-transfer of cells to the donor of the protective graft, tolerance of the graft to antigens of the original host persisted [ZAALBERG and VAN DER MEUL, 1966]. Tolerance persists even if the secondary host has been preimmunized against cells of the primary host. Cellular chimaerism was thus not a prerequisite for maintaining tolerance in this system.

The tolerance to erythrocytes proved to be a much more suitable model for analysing the role of antigen in maintaining the tolerant state. MITCHISON [1959, 1962 a, 1962 b] studied this in chickens in a model of tolerance to homologous erythrocytes. As has already been stated, chickens are excellent producers of antibodies against homologous erythrocytes. Chickens injected with homologous erythrocytes practically always form antibodies against them. Survival in the circulation of erythrocytes labelled with radioactive chromium appeared to be a very sensitive test for the presence of these antibodies in the circulation. The elimination of homologous erythrocytes is regularly accelerated in chickens as a result of antibody formation. Since erythrocytes have a limited life-span and are unable to divide, their injection cannot induce permanent chimaerism in the recipient's body which might become a permanent source of antigen. However, erythrocytes are difficult to separate from white blood cells, which can cause the development of chimaerism. To exclude this possibility MITCHISON irradiated the blood used for the injections with 10000 r. This irradiation dose blocked the production of white blood cells but did not influence the survival of red blood cells. MITCHISON induced tolerance by injections of blood given before and/or after hatching. Labelling with radioactive chromium permitted a simple and accurate quantitative determination of the course of survival of injected erythrocytes. When erythrocytes began to disappear from the circulation, further injections were given and the procedure was repeated. Tolerance induced was generally incomplete. The tolerated erythrocytes survived longer than non-tolerated ones, but shorter than autologous erythrocytes. In spite of its incompleteness, tolerance induced lasted almost indefinitely when the injections were continued. When they were stopped, tolerance disappeared, but the interval between the cessation of the injection series and the loss of tolerance, i. e., the onset of immune elimination of previously tolerated erythrocytes, varied from less than 5 days to over 215 days. The interval increased with the age of the animal. The same results were obtained by HAŠEK in a similar model in a heterologous system [HAŠEK, 1960]. Even here the interval between the interruption in the supply of antigen and the disappearance of tolerance was extended with increasing age [HAŠEK, 1963 b, 1965 a, 1965 b].

The antigen injections were started in these experiments in the perinatal period; therefore the total dosage of antigen was greater and exposure to antigen longer in animals which were older at the time when administration of antigen was discontinued, compared with younger animals. All these three factors might cause a prolonged duration of tolerance, but from the materials presented it could not be determined which factor(s) might be responsible. Evidence that tolerance disappears more rapidly in young than in older animals was provided by MITCHISON with mice paralysed with BSA, where the factor of the difference between the dosage of antigen and the length of exposure to antigen was eliminated [MITCHISON, 1965]. This relationship was also supported by our results with tolerance to HSA in young and adult mature chickens. Using the same dose we found it was more difficult to induce tolerance in young adults, which also lost tolerance more rapidly, than in mature adults [IVÁNYI et al., 1964 a]. A quantitative comparison was, however, difficult in our experiments owing to a more rapid catabolism of HSA in young chickens [IVÁNYI et al., 1964 b].

Evidence of the dependence of tolerance on the presence of antigen in the body seemed to be so convincing that this requirement was included into the definition of tolerance as a prerequisite of its permanency [MEDAWAR, 1962]. SMITH and BRIDGES [1958] calculated that at the time when tolerance was disappearing in rabbits, 10^{12}–10^{13} molecules of antigen were still present in their circulation. This might suggest the possibility that this pool of antigen plays a decisive role in maintaining tolerance. On the other hand, MITCHISON's observations

[1962 b] that, after the cessation of erythrocyte injections into chickens, tolerance persisted in some cases for a multiple of the life-span of erythrocytes are at variance with this assumption. Further findings also cast some doubt on the possibility of drawing categorical conclusions in this respect. Bussard [1962] and Humphrey [1964 a] observed that tolerance to heterologous serum proteins persisted in some rabbits although, if the experiments had turned out according to expectation, the antigen should have been completely eliminated from their circulation. Interesting results were obtained with tolerance in turkeys and ducks toward chicken erythrocyte antigens which determined the susceptibility of adult animals in these species to the development of tumours induced by Rous sarcoma virus [Svoboda and Hašek, 1956; Svoboda, 1958, 1966; Hašek et al., 1963]. Tolerance to this antigen persists for a long time, though neither complete tolerance to chicken erythrocytes nor a decrease in haemagglutinin formation is detectable and, moreover, natural heteroagglutinins against chicken erythrocytes are present in tolerant animals. That tolerance in this case does not depend on cellular chimaerism has been further confirmed by the finding that tolerance leading to the development of Rous sarcoma could be induced even by lyophilized chicken cells.

Thus it has not been confirmed that cellular chimaerism or the presence of antigen in the circulation are essential for the maintenance of tolerance. Neither do the findings obtained provide evidence against the claim that the presence of antigen at some site outside the circulation might be an absolute prerequisite for the persistence of tolerance. The methods of detection of antigen are not sensitive enough, and therefore very little is known about the localization and fate of the antigen. In a study of tolerance to BSA in mice Mitchison [1965] found that it persisted after the antigen had been eliminated from the circulation, but the loss of tolerance coincided with the disappearance of antigen which persisted intracellularly in a detectable form. This is the only finding so far and it is not certain whether the disappearance of antigen is in fact the cause of the loss of tolerance and, if this is so, whether this finding is generally valid. I assume therefore that the failure to demonstrate the presence of antigen in the body of the individual who is specifically unresponsive to it for a long time should not be the reason against not regarding this state as immunological tolerance when it possesses its other features. If this argument is adopted, then the inclusion of the Sulzberger-Chase phenomenon with the tolerant states will not raise any difficulties.

(g) The Sulzberger-Chase Phenomenon

This is the longest-known tolerance phenomenon; it was described in the late 1920's as having been observed in humans and guinea-pigs. FREI [1928] observed that intravenous injections of Neosalvarsan administered to patients suffering from syphilis rendered them unable to develop skin sensitivity to the same chemical. Similar results were obtained experimentally by SULZBERGER [1929 a, 1929 b] in guinea-pigs. Independently of these findings, CHASE [1946] discovered that the ability of guinea-pigs to become sensitized with simple chemicals could be suppressed by the peroral administration of the respective allergen prior to sensitization. Suppression produced in this way was specific and applied to both skin hypersensitivity of the delayed type and formation of circulating antibodies, at least when elicited by immunization with the respective allergen bound to guinea-pig serum proteins. The central character of the immunological suppression was demonstrated with the Sulzberger-Chase phenomenon as early as the 1940's [CHASE, 1949] by the adoptive transfer of lymphoid cells. In unresponsive animals neither blocking nor inhibiting antibodies could be detected, and non-reactivity could be suppressed by the adoptive transfer of cells from an immune animal.

Although the suppression persisted for a very long time, the retention of allergen by which it had been induced could not be detected in the body over this time [BATTISTO and CHASE, 1963]. As has been emphasized in the concluding parts of the preceding paragraph, I do not regard this as a prerequisite for classifying a certain phenomenon as immunological tolerance. As the first volume of this series of monographs dealt with the Sulzberger-Chase phenomenon [DE WECK and FREY, 1966] I will not refer to it unless it is of special relevance to the elucidation of more general problems of immunological tolerance.

2. Central Failure of the Mechanism of Immunological Response in Immunological Tolerance

In the preceding chapter I was concerned with the states of immunological inhibition that are regarded as immunological tolerance. Immunological tolerance is a suppression state of the immune reaction due to specific central failure of the mechanism of immunological response. However, there are specific suppression

states of the immune reaction indistinguishable from immunological
tolerance in their manifestations, which are brought about by a different mechanism. It is possible that some of them may be due to a central
failure of the mechanism of the immune reaction which is, however,
mediated by the action of antibodies on immunologically competent
cells. The concept and the definition of immunological tolerance do
not presume that these forms of suppression might be regarded as
tolerance. In immunological tolerance, the central failure should be
the primary one brought about by a direct, non-mediated action of
antigen just as the antigen induces by its direct action an immune reaction [Medawar, 1962]. Before embarking on the analysis of evidence bearing on the extent to which this mechanism in immunological tolerance is a verified fact and the extent to which it is a hypothesis, I would like to describe briefly three specific inhibition states
which are known and in one case at least presumed to be due to a
mechanism other than immunological tolerance.

(a) Immunosuppression by Humoral Antibodies

Abundant evidence has been accumulated in immunological literature
that the presence of circulating antibodies, either actively formed by
the recipient or passively introduced to him, may reduce specifically
antibody formation against the respective antigen. This question has
been studied in detail by Uhr and Bauman [1961] with diphtheria
toxoid, BSA, BGG and ovalbumin in guinea-pigs and rabbits. Antibodies were mainly introduced in the form of a specific precipitate
with antigen, but also separately from antigen. Antitoxin given as late
as 5 days after the injection of antigen was found to be still capable of
inhibiting antibody formation. This finding seems to be at variance
with the view that the suppression observed is due to an afferent blocking of the antigenic stimulus by antibodies, as a result of which the
antigen cannot reach the cells responsible for an immune reaction.
When the antibody is introduced a relatively long time after the injection of antigen, then the antigen may stimulate the immune response.
This fact was explained by assuming that the antigen was needed
for permanent synthesis of antibodies. If the antigen is bound even at
a time when the immune reaction has started, then its absence would
stop further antibody formation.

    This view has to be somewhat modified in the light of the findings
of Möller and Wigzell [1965], who produced suppression of the

immune reaction of mice toward sheep erythrocytes by means of anti-bodies against this antigen. The method of localized haemolysis in gel permitted the study of the course of the immune reaction in this system, not only by detecting circulating antibodies but also by determining the number of cells forming 19S haemolysins. Antibodies introduced later than antigen did not decrease the number of antibody-forming cells already present at the time of serum injection, but blocked a further increase in their number. The formation of 19S antibodies could be inhibited much more easily by means of 7S than 19S anti-bodies. There was a 100–200-fold difference in their effectiveness. As regards the nature of antibodies, the situation is similar to that observed in suppression of the immune response against phage $\varnothing$ X 174 [FINKELSTEIN and UHR, 1964].

These findings led to the assumption that 7S antibodies might act as a feed-back mechanism for 19S antibody formation. The possibility of inhibiting 7S antibody formation against sheep erythrocytes by means of passively introduced antibodies was also demonstrated later at the level of both circulating antibodies and antibody-forming cells [WIGZELL, 1966]. The efficacy of this inhibition decreased with the time elapsed from immunization, but could be demonstrated even if antibodies were introduced as late as 40 days after immunization. In this case, as in inhibition of 19S antibody formation, the production of 7S antibodies was not inhibited in cells which were already producing them. The 7S antibodies may therefore probably also act as a feed-back mechanism for their own production. If they play such a role in this regulation, then their effect is much smaller here than on 19S antibody formation.

ROWLEY and FITCH [1964] found that the formation of antibodies against sheep erythrocytes could be inhibited by introducing anti-bodies either to X-irradiated recipients, to which cells from untreated donors were transferred, or directly to donors. The inhibition was obtained even if the transferred cells were incubated in vitro with the respective antiserum. This is difficult to explain by assuming that passively introduced antibodies act at the afferent level by binding the antigen, and in contrast, the view is supported that they act centrally, directly on lymphoid cells responsible for the immune reaction.

However, in the system of antibody formation against flagellar antigen of S. adelaide it was impossible to induce the inhibition by specific antiserum when this was incubated in vitro with lymphoid cells transferred to irradiated recipients. In this system no inhibition of the immune response could be induced even when antiserum was injected into cell donors before the transfer to irradiated recipients. The only effective way was the binding of antibodies to bacteria *in vitro* prior to their inoculation [Möller, 1964 b].

On the other hand, the possibility that this kind of immune suppression can be the result of a direct action of antibodies on cells seems to be supported by the finding that much higher doses of antibodies bound to injected erythrocytes are needed to obtain the same suppression effect on the immune reaction to heterologous erythrocytes than when antiserum was injected to immunized animals separately from antigen [Merchant, 1966; personal communication]. This mode of action of antibodies is, however, opposed by the finding that antibodies devoid of F_c fragment do not lose their capacity to inhibit the immune reaction to the phage ØX 174 [Tao and Uhr, 1966]. Since this portion of the molecule plays a role in the fixation of antibodies to the skin, it seems likely, though not certain, that this portion should be of decisive importance for the interaction of antibodies with lymphoid cells. These contradictory findings were made on different experimental models, so that the possibility is not excluded that there is a different mechanism of action of antibodies in different systems.

(b) Immune Deviation

This is a specific suppression of the immune reaction caused by the prior injection of antigen. The phenomenon has been described in guinea-pigs [Asherson and Stone, 1965], in which the injection of various heterologous proteins in complete Freund's adjuvant leads to delayed-type hypersensitivity besides the production of circulating antibodies. If the same antigen is injected in an alum-precipitated form before the injection in complete Freund's adjuvant and sometimes even after that, the delayed hypersensitivity reaction is reduced. A similar effect can also be obtained using a soluble antigen or antigen in incomplete Freund's adjuvant [Asherson and Stone, 1965; Dvorak et al., 1965, 1966; Dvorak and Flax, 1966; Loewi et al., 1966]. The total amount of circulating antibodies produced after immunization in complete Freund's adjuvant was practically the same in both groups or was higher in animals treated in this way than in the untreated ones. A detailed analysis showed that the formation of γ_2-antibodies was reduced whereas the formation of γ_1-antibodies was not suppressed in pretreated animals. This inhibition of immune reaction is specific, as it applies only to the antigen used for the induction of immune deviation.

Of particular importance for the understanding of the mechanism of immune deviation was the discovery that in these models the induction of delayed hypersensitivity could not be prevented by the passive transfer of serum [LOEWI et al., 1966; ASHERSON, 1966]. It is, however, not certain whether these results can be regarded as fully conclusive. If antibodies turn out to be effective in the transfer of immune deviation, then this would be an example of immunosuppression caused by antibodies where the specific cell hypersensitivity and not production of circulating antibodies is inhibited. As the present evidence is against this view, let us assume that the mechanism of immune deviation is different and that it is induced by a direct action of antigen.

If this is the case, then the question arises how the mechanism of this inhibition caused by direct action of antigen, not mediated through another immune reaction, differs from that of immunological tolerance. Would the cells responsible for different types of immune reaction be of common origin, then the antigen introduced for the induction of immune deviation might activate a portion of cells from the reservoir available for the immune reaction and might determine them for γ_1-antibody formation. These cells would then be pre-empted and would no longer be available for delayed hypersensitivity and formation of γ_2-antibodies. This may be the cause of the lower intensity of such reactions in deviated animals.

It is, however, far from impossible that cells of different origin are responsible for the different types of immune reaction. In this case, it is not easy to imagine which type of their reciprocal specific interaction might be involved, and the problem of identity or disparity of the mechanisms engaged in immune deviation and tolerance is of decisive importance. The findings that the inhibition of all types of immune reaction, which would probably better correspond to the concepts of immunological tolerance, may be achieved by higher doses of antigen than immune deviation [ASHERSON and STONE, 1965; WEIGLE, 1966a] cannot be used as an argument against the identity of the mechanism of both these inhibitions. Different amounts of antigen could be required for the induction of immunological tolerance in each type of immune reaction: the lowest amount would be needed for delayed hypersensitivity, a higher amount for γ_2-antibodies and the highest amount for γ_1-antibodies. The identity of the mechanism of immune deviation and of tolerance is, however, opposed by the fact that the deviation can be induced by alum-precipitated antigen or antigen incorporated in incomplete Freund's adjuvant, whereas a soluble antigen seems to be needed for the induction of tolerance.

The question of the mechanism of immune deviation still remains open. This makes it difficult to decide whether certain phenomena may be included in this category. For example, it has been shown by Boyden [1957] that the injection of unheated tuberculoprotein eliciting the appearance of circulating antibodies retarded the development of delayed hypersensitivity to tuberculin, when given prior to the inoculation of live BCG. Circulating antibodies were present on the 11th day after the injection of BCG in treated animals, but not in the untreated control group vaccinated with BCG. A similar observation was made by Arima et al. [1958]. The development of tuberculin hypersensitivity in guinea-pigs experimentally infected with *Mycob. tuberculosis* was delayed by the intravenous injection of live or killed bacteria of various human strains of this species given simultaneously with or after the infecting inoculum. The avian strain had no such effects. Both these phenomena may be caused by immune deviation.

(c) Immunological Enhancement

Allogeneic tumour grafts are rejected in the same manner as grafts of normal tissues. As a rule, transplantation immunity of the recipient to individual antigens of the tumour is fully responsible for their rejection. The tumour has the same antigens as the animal in which the tumour originated. The transplantation immune reaction against a specific tumour antigen is not significant in allotransplantation [Koldovský, 1967]. The survival of some tumours in allogeneic hosts has been made possible by injecting the recipient with lyophilized or otherwise killed tissues of the donor strain before transplantation of the tumour. In this way, the survival of the tumour could be so prolonged as to kill the host. This phenomenon has been called immunological enhancement. It has been widely studied in mice, but has also been observed in other animal species. Immunological enhancement has been induced not only to individual antigens of the tumour in histoincompatible recipients, but also to specific tumour antigens within inbred strains. Immunological enhancement is confined not only to tumour but also to normal tissue grafts [Billingham et al., 1956b; Brent and Medawar, 1961; Nelson, 1962; Möller, 1964a]. However, the prolongation in the survival of normal tissues is relatively short here and is of no practical significance for overcoming tissue incompatibility. The marked difference in the survival of normal tissue and tumour grafts is, to some extent, an optical illusion. While a small prolongation in the survival of normal tissue grafts does not alter the fate of the graft, the same small advantage makes the tumour grafts grow progressively until death of the host. Thus the whole situation is essentially changed. Instead of rejection of an allogeneic graft, the tumour graft kills the host. The dividing line between death of the graft and death of the host has been passed here. An important factor which makes the progressive growth of the tumour in immuno-logical enhancement possible is its lesser susceptibility to transplanta-tion immunity. Transplantation tolerance can also make possible the growth of tumours in an otherwise incompatible host [KOPROWSKI, 1955]. The tumour grafts are more suitable for testing incomplete transplantation tolerance. Their advantage obviously does not hold good with the states of strong tolerance, where even the grafts of normal tissues survive much longer and sometimes permanently. In contrast, progressive tumour growth causing the death of the host may reduce the time over which tolerance can be tested. However, the states of weak transplantation tolerance that might not be manifest, or might escape detection by means of normal tissue grafts, can be re-vealed by tumour tissue grafts. It is especially advantageous to use xenogeneic tumour grafts for detecting transplantation tolerance in interspecific relationships, which is, as a rule, weak [BOLLAG, 1955].

Of paramount importance in understanding the mechanism of immunological enhancement was the discovery that enhancement could be transferred to untreated recipients by serum from animals injected with tissue lyophilisates. The use of lyophilized or otherwise devitalized tissues for immunization is not a prerequisite for obtaining the respective type of antibodies. The serum from animals that had acquired transplantation immunity after graft rejection can also be effective [KALISS, 1956]. On the other hand, the lyophilized tissue used for the induction of tolerance also induces transplantation im-munity [HAŠKOVÁ and SVOBODA, 1962; HAŠKOVÁ et al., 1962]. The important point is the fact that immunological enhancement is me-diated through an immune reaction elicited by active or passive immunization.

Immunological enhancement was thought to be due to a change in tumour cells brought about by antibodies whereby their sensitivity to transplantation immunity was altered [KALISS, 1958, 1962; FELD-

MAN and GLOBERSON, 1960]. Although such an alteration may occur, it is not a general phenomenon [SNELL et al., 1960; MÖLLER, 1963b] and might not cause the rapid change in behaviour which takes place, for example, when the enhancing antiserum is given after the injection of a tumour inoculum.

The enhancing antibodies thus evidently interfere with the course of transplantation immunity. The induction of enhancement in untreated recipients using tumour cells to which the enhancing antibodies are attached [MÖLLER, 1963b] suggests that the interference takes place at the peripheral level of the host's immune reaction. The reduction of the transplantation immune reaction in enhanced recipients [SNELL et al., 1960; BRENT and MEDAWAR, 1961] might result from blocking the afferent part of the immune reaction. The possibility cannot be excluded that antibodies act directly on lymphoid cells responsible for the immune reaction. However, this has not been proved even in better defined systems, as is stated in the preceding paragraph.

Finally, the cases of antagonism between different immune reactions to the same antigen at the efferent level are worth considering. CHUTNÁ and RYCHLÍKOVÁ [1964b] studied the cytotoxic damage to guinea-pig testicular cells by antibodies formed in guinea-pigs after immunization with testicular antigen in complete Freund's adjuvant. No damage was observed when testicular cells were incubated with serum from guinea-pigs immunized with testicular antigens in saline without adjuvant prior to exposure to the cytotoxic antibodies. This method of immunization produced no cytotoxins, but antibodies detectable by PCA reaction. The latter seem to be an effective agent preventing the damage to cells by cytotoxic antibodies. A similar competition at the level of effectors of the cellular and humoral type seems also to exist in immunological enhancement [MÖLLER, 1963c].

It is not known which fraction of antibodies is responsible for the enhancing activity [KALISS and KANDUTSCH, 1956; BUBENÍK et al., 1965; VOISIN et al., 1966; HAŠEK et al., 1966b]. Neither is it known against which form of cellular individual antigen the enhancing antibodies are directed. From what has been said it seems likely that the enhancing antibodies may act at different levels of the immune reaction and that the mechanism of their action may be different at different levels. Lastly, it is not certain whether the prolongation in the graft survival produced by immunization with tissue lyophilisates may be limited to the action of the enhancing antibodies, and whether other mechanisms, e.g., immune deviation may also be involved.

(d) Suppression of Various Forms of Immune Reaction in Immunological Tolerance

BURNET and FENNER's original concept of immunological tolerance as a process of recognition of tolerated antigen as an indigenous substance, against which the tolerant animal does not react, implies that all immune reactions to a tolerated antigen should be suppressed. In recent years, the knowledge of various types of immune response has extended considerably, and it is really surprising how many of these types can be induced by immunization with a single antigen. The most complete data relative to the inhibition of all immune reactions in immunological tolerance have been accumulated in studies of the Sulzberger-Chase phenomenon. In this state, not only contact dermatitis due to delayed hypersensitivity, but also the formation of γ_1- and γ_2-antibodies has been shown to be suppressed [CHASE, 1963; BATTISTO and BLOOM, 1966]. Similar evidence is available for tolerance to heterologous proteins. In guinea-pigs rendered tolerant of BSA or HGG in the perinatal period, both formation of the circulating antibodies responsible for the elimination of antigen and for anaphylaxis and delayed hypersensitivity were suppressed [HUMPHREY and TURK, 1961; TURK and HUMPHREY, 1961]. Similarly, delayed hypersensitivity and formation of antibodies responsible for PCA were suppressed in guinea-pigs made tolerant by an intrauterine injection of ovalbumin [GREGG and SALVIN, 1963]. Also in rabbits rendered tolerant of HSA shortly after birth, both delayed hypersensitivity and also formation of the antibodies which cause an immediate reaction in skin tests and of those which are responsible for the precipitation reaction and for the elimination of antigen from the circulation, were suppressed [CHUTNÁ and HRABA, 1962]. In these experiments for detection of delayed hypersensitivity an HSA precipitate with rabbit anti-HSA antibodies was used [LESKOWITZ, 1960]. We proved the specificity of this method of detection of delayed hypersensitivity by the transfer of lymphoid cells or serum from rabbits immunized with HSA in complete Freund's adjuvant to non-immune recipients.

In some cases, only some forms of immune reaction are suppressed while others persist. For example, it has been shown by TURK and HUMPHREY [1961] that while delayed hypersensitivity and antibody formation were suppressed in most of the guinea-pigs which had been rendered tolerant by the injection of heterologous protein at a very early age, one group of animals treated with HGG which did not display delayed hypersensitivity toward this antigen was capable of producing circulating antibodies against it. Borel *et al.* [1966] were successful in suppressing delayed hypersensitivity, but not the formation of circulating antibodies in newborn guinea-pigs when injecting them with DNP-BGG. Finally, Battisto and Chase [1965] were able to elicit the formation of circulating antibodies by immunization with hapten bound to a heterologous protein carrier in animals rendered tolerant of this hapten by its peroral administration. The animals, however, remained non-reactive when tested for contact hypersensitivity.

The results of Turk and Humphrey and of Battisto and Chase were obtained from models in which complete tolerance can be induced, i.e., both these forms of immune reaction can be suppressed. The suppression of delayed hypersensitivity while circulating antibodies are produced seems to be evidence that in these experiments incomplete tolerance was induced. The same is probably true in the experiments of Borel *et al.* [1966]. It can be seen from this that the suppression of delayed hypersensitivity is easier to induce, or disappears later than the suppression of circulating antibody production.

The difference in inducibility of immunological tolerance has also been observed with other types of immune reactions. In newborn animals [Nossal, 1966] and in adults in which antimetabolites were used [Borel *et al.*, 1965; Sahiar and Schwartz, 1965; Blinkoff, 1966] it appeared that the formation of 7 S antibody could be more readily suppressed than that of 19 S antibody. The agreement in the ease with induction of the suppression of delayed hypersensitivity and formation of circulating antibodies between immunological tolerance and immune deviation is surprising. It would be of interest to learn whether a similar agreement will be observed in immune reactions giving rise to formation of various types of circulating antibodies. In immune deviation the formation of γ_2-antibodies can be suppressed, whereas the formation of γ_1-antibodies remains unchanged, or may even be increased. However, relevant data are not available in a comparable model for immunological tolerance.

The present evidence therefore supports the view that in complete tolerance all types of immune response are really suppressed. There are cases of tolerant states where only some types of immune reaction are suppressed, but in the same models it has been shown that all types of such reactions may be inhibited. This makes it unlikely that incomplete suppression in the cases mentioned might be caused by a mechanism other than immunological tolerance. This conclusion is not firmly established; even if it were true, it would be difficult to say that other mechanisms, e. g., immunosuppression through circulating antibodies, or immune deviation, do not participate in bringing about the suppression. For this reason it is much easier to study the nature of the mechanism of immune inhibition in tolerance in the states where tolerance is complete.

(e) Evidence on Central Character of Immunological Inhibition in Immunological Tolerance

The first objection raised against the view that central inhibition is the cause of immunological tolerance was based on the hypothesis that only masking of the immune reaction by an excess of the antigen in the body might be involved [KAPLAN et al., 1950]. This objection may best be applied in immunological paralysis and transplantation tolerance. In the chapters dealing with different types of the tolerant state evidence has been presented against this explanation of their mechanism by means of the adoptive transfer of lymphoid cells from non-tolerant animals. The possibility of accomplishing the immune reaction to a tolerated antigen by transferred lymphoid cells in the tolerant organism appears to be a good argument against this view. As the adoptive transfer is not a very sensitive method for demonstrating an immune reaction [MÄKELÄ and MITCHISON, 1965 a], this evidence is convincing.

Another objection raised against the presumed mechanism of immunological tolerance was based on the hypothesis that an inhibition brought about by antibodies is actually involved [ROWLEY and FITCH, 1965 a, 1965 b]. The demonstration of the absence of antibody formation by serological methods generally has a relatively high threshold level of sensitivity. The inhibition of antibody formation can be achieved by very small quantities of antibodies escaping serological detection. Of much importance to the solution of this question was the finding that in tolerant animals an immune reaction cannot be demonstrated even at the level of antibody-forming cells [SERCARZ and COONS, 1959, 1963]. These authors tried to detect such cells in immunological paralysis and tolerance to proteins in mice by immuno-fluorescence. The absence of antibody-forming cells which they observed in both these states was direct evidence that tolerance was complete, and supported the view that these states are due to central inhibition of the immune response. They carried out these experiments to prove that in these states masking of antibody formation by an excess of the tolerated antigen in the organism is not involved. Their results furnished conclusive support for this claim as well as evidence against the above hypothesis that tolerance is the result of immuno-suppression by circulating antibodies. If antibody formation were responsible for the suppression, then the antibody-forming cells should be detected by this method. The significance of these con-clusions is unfortunately limited by the small screening capacity of the method used. An ideal method in this respect seems to be the method of localized haemolysis in gel [JERNE and NORDIN, 1963; INGRAHAM and BUSSARD, 1964]. By this method even small numbers of antibody-forming cells can be detected in large cell populations. In its original form only 19S haemolytic antibodies against erythrocytes could be detected. The limitation due to the nature of antibodies could be removed, to a large extent, by using an anti-gamma globulin serum for the detection of antibody-forming cells without or with low haemolytic activity probably of the 7S type [DRESSER and WORTIS, 1965; ŠTERZL and ŘÍHA, 1965]. In most experiments using the method of localized haemolysis in gel, heterologous erythrocytes served as the detecting antigen. They are, however, scarcely suitable for elucidating the question of the central suppression in immunological tolerance because, as a rule, only partial tolerance towards them can be induced. Only the use of homologous erythrocytes recently described [HILDE-MANN and PINKERTON, 1966; MCBRIDE and SCHIERMAN, 1966] offers the possibility of studying more suitable systems of this kind.

The limitation caused by erythrocyte antigens used as a detection system was avoided by using erythrocytes with passively bound anti-gens. The first antigen used with success was bacterial endotoxin [LANDY et al., 1965]. Another suitable material was simple chemical haptens coupled to erythrocytes [HRABA and MERCHANT, 1966; MER-CHANT and HRABA, 1966]. In this model attempts were made to demonstrate antibody-forming cells in the tolerant animals [MER-CHANT et al., 1967]. Tolerance was induced in rabbits by injections of sulphanil-BSA starting from the first day after birth. To ensure com-plete tolerance to the carrier, the treated rabbits were injected with

100 mg BSA on the 6th day and with 20 mg on the 26th day. The rabbits were killed after challenge at the age of 12 weeks. In all 15 control rabbits from the same litters the circulating antibodies against sulphanilic acid and the carrier protein were detectable in serum and large numbers of cells forming 19S and 7S antibodies against sulphanilic acid in the spleen. Of the 17 treated animals, only 2 contained significant numbers of cells forming antibodies against sulphanilic acid. Circulating antibodies were detected in only one of these two reactive rabbits. In the other treated animals circulating antibodies could not be found. The number of cells forming plaques by means of 19S haemolysins was slightly higher to sulphanil-erythrocytes in these animals than to the carriers alone. The difference is significant (P < 0.02), but it is not certain whether cells forming antibodies against sulphanilic acid are in fact involved. The difference may be only the result of a higher sensitivity of conjugated erythrocytes to the lysis by antibodies against the carrier erythrocytes. A follow-up of cells forming plaques by means of 7S antibodies did not reveal any significant difference in the number of plaques between labelled erythrocytes and the background. This is strong evidence against the view that immunological inhibition might be due to immuno-suppression by antibodies as effective antibodies are of the 7S type.

Thus none of the present findings on the nature of the suppression of immunological reactivity in immunological tolerance is in disagreement with the concept that it is due to a primary central failure of the mechanism of immunological reaction, as has been postulated in the definition. The only reservation I would make results from the fact that the evidence available is based on the demonstration of the absence of immune reactions. Each of these demonstrations, at the effector level or at the level of antibody-forming cells, has a certain threshold level of sensitivity. Only the absence of immune reaction above this threshold level can be detected. The conclusion that inhibition of such immune reactions is complete in tolerance is therefore likely, but cannot be supported by direct evidence; below the threshold level of sensitivity of the methods used our supposition of the absence of immune reactions remains hypothetical. It is questionable, but could be subjected to analysis, whether such a minimal immune reaction might be instrumental in causing immune suppression. The findings of MERCHANT et al. [1967] do not favour this possibility.

(f) Partial Tolerance

By partial tolerance we understand a state of inhibition of immune reaction manifesting itself not as complete suppression of the immune reaction, but as a decrease in its intensity; this state is either induced by antigen applied in the same way as for induction of complete tolerance in similar situations, or succeeds the state of complete tolerance.

A typical example of partial tolerance is reduced antibody formation which can be achieved in chickens by the intraembryonic administration of foreign erythrocytes [SIMONSEN, 1955; HAŠEK and HRABA, 1955a] (Fig.1) or by the injection of heterologous serum proteins before or shortly after hatching [WOLFE et al., 1957; STEVENS et al., 1958]. An example of the other way in which partial tolerance arises is reduced antibody formation against heterologous serum proteins in rabbits after complete tolerance induced at birth has disappeared [HUMPHREY, 1964b]. A further example of partial tolerance is prolongation, but not permanent survival, of skin grafts towards which tolerance has been induced in very young animals [BILLINGHAM et al., 1956a].

The state of partial tolerance is interesting because of the possibilities offered for its analysis. In complete tolerance, all the methods

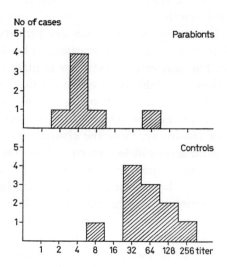

Fig. 1. Titres of immune agglutinins against chicken erythrocytes in ducks, embryonic parabionts with chickens [after HAŠEK and HRABA, 1955b].

available for the study of immune reactions serve to confirm, on the basis of negative findings obtained, that the state of tolerance is complete and that it is not caused by any immune reaction. On the other hand, partial tolerance is open to positive analysis by these methods because of the presence of immune reactions.

Before attempting to summarize the findings obtained by this analysis, I would like to pay attention to the concepts of the cellular background of immunological tolerance. In principle, there are two possibilities how this state is realized at the cellular level. One possibility is the elimination of cells capable of immune reaction to a tolerated antigen. A second possibility is the retention of these cells and inhibition of their capacity for immune reaction. The instructive theory of antibody formation does not mean a choice between these two possibilities; if the antigen can instruct any immunologically competent cell for the formation of specific antibodies, then the elimination of all these cells would result in total suppression of immune reactions, i.e., non-specific inhibition of immunological reactivity. If the instructive theory were true, then the specific elimination of reactivity must take place at a subcellular level.

The selective hypothesis of antibody formation leaves the way open for both these mechanisms. In the original formulation of the clonal selection hypothesis it has been postulated that tolerance is realized by the destruction of the clone capable of immune reactions to the tolerated antigen. Instead of a physical elimination, the functional elimination can be admitted when cells of this clone temporarily or permanently lose the capability of immune reaction though they are not destroyed. The presence of such a mute clone is then functionally indistinguishable from its absence.

The question of whether tolerance is due to the absence of cells capable of the respective immune reaction or to their inhibition is, however, essential from a theoretical point of view. In the first case, tolerance is a property of the whole organism, i.e. of its lymphoid system as a whole, while in the second case, tolerance is a property of the individual cells. Unfortunately, no method is available for the demonstration of tolerant cells, just as we cannot identify immunologically competent cells that do not form antibodies. In the case of partial tolerance the question arises whether the reduction in antibody formation is due to a lower production of antibodies by individual cells, the number of which is approximately the same in tolerant and non-tolerant animals, or whether it is the result of a lower number of these

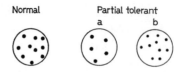

Fig. 2. Hypotheses explaining partial tolerance at the cellular level. – (a) Partial tolerance caused by a lower number of antibody-forming cells as compared with normal individuals. The quantity of antibody produced by one cell is the same in partially tolerant and control animals. (b) Partially tolerant cells exist. They produce less antibody than normal cells. The number of antibody-forming cells is the same in partially tolerant and normal individuals.

cells in tolerant animals (Fig.2). The finding of the existence of partially tolerant cells would be an indirect, but very strong support for the view that tolerance is due to the existence of tolerant cells.

Attempts were made to answer this question in rats which were rendered tolerant of sheep erythrocytes by a series of injections starting from birth [HAŠEK *et al.*, 1965, 1966]. Two groups of animals were used as controls: one group was given only the immunizing dose of antigen, and the other group received two injections of antigen spaced 10 days apart. In the tolerant group the titres of haemolysins were lower than in the two control groups. The highest titres were noted in the control group given only one immunizing dose. The group given two injections of sheep erythrocytes gave lower titres than the first group. The number of cells forming haemolysins was determined by the method of localized haemolysis in gel in ŠTERZL's modification [ŠTERZL *et al.*, 1965]. Their number was the lowest in tolerant animals and in the other groups it rose in parallel to increasing antibody titre (Fig.3). A rough correlation between the titre of circulating antibodies and the number of plaque-forming cells also did not indicate the possibility of a lower antibody production by individual cells of tolerant animals. These results clearly showed that in these animals partial tolerance was not due to the existence of partially tolerant cells, but to a lower number of antibody-forming cells. Similar results were obtained in mice by FRIEDMAN [1965a] using a similar model.

The most serious objection to this experiment is that repeated injections of sheep erythrocytes have stimulated 7S antibody formation which may display the inhibitory effects on the formation of 19S antibody. Reduction in the number of antibody-forming cells in pre-

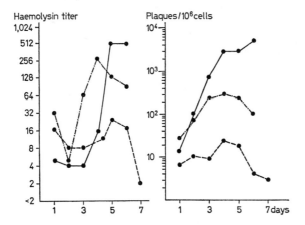

Fig. 3. Haemolysin titres and numbers of plaque-forming cells in rats partially tolerant to sheep erythrocytes and in normal rats. ------- = tolerant group; ———— = non-preimmunized control group; –·–·–·– = preimmunized control group; x = days after challenge; y = serum dilution or number of plaque-forming cells per 10^6 spleen cells [after Hašek *et al.*, 1965].

sumably tolerant animals would actually be the outcome of immuno-suppression by antibodies.

Therefore in further experiments, we looked for 7S plaque-forming cells. We found, that their number was significantly lower in the tolerant than in the control groups. The data obtained therefore confirm for both types of antibody-forming cells that partial tolerance is associated with their lower numbers.

Unfortunately, the conclusion that the existence of partially tolerant cells could not be proved leaves open too many possibilities in explaining the mechanism of tolerance at a cellular level. These findings agree with the original concept of the clonal theory of antibody formation. If tolerance is the absence of the clone capable of forming a certain antibody, then when this clone appears there is no reason why its cells should produce less antibody. On the other hand, the findings presented do not exclude the possibility that the tolerant cells do exist, but their shift into a reactive state may have the nature of an all-or-nothing process. The only clue is given by the fact that partial tolerance may be a long-persisting state. This means that the lower number of antibody-forming cells can be maintained over a relatively long period of time and that the tolerant organism is not capable of increasing their number. This situation may be best explained by assuming that the proliferation of cells reacting with a tolerated antigen is blocked by the tolerant cells which can compete with the reactive cells for the space. This argument is, however, not very strong at the present state of knowledge of the mechanisms regulating the cell relations. Moreover, it is not clear whether the model studied really involves partial tolerance, i.e., lower reactivity to the same antigens, or split-tolerance, i.e., complete tolerance towards some erythrocyte antigens and normal reactivity to the others. Then the above findings at the cellular level would not be at all surprising. The number of antibody-forming cells would be lower, because less of the erythrocyte antigens would evoke an immune response.

The existence of partial tolerance in this sense has not yet been demonstrated unequivocally in any model. The states of tolerance to defined antigens that are chemical units are known to exist where the production of antibodies against these antigens is reduced. An example may be tolerance to heterologous serum proteins in chickens. These substances, in spite of being chemical units, possess several different antigenic determinants. It is unlikely that antibodies against all these individual determinants are mostly or even exclusively formed by one cell. If the production of antibodies against different determinants were confined to different cell clones, then split-tolerance might easily occur at the level of the determinants of the same macromolecule. There is no great hope of answering this question by means of a simple hapten when the nature of its carrier will not ensure that it will form with the given hapten only one type of antigenic determinant. Unless this is elucidated, the problem of the cellular background of partial tolerance cannot be solved conclusively.

3. The Relationship
between Immunity and Immunological Tolerance

(a) Immune Reaction during Induction of Tolerance

According to the original hypothesis of immunological tolerance, the possibility of its induction exists only in the early stages of individual development when the lymphoid system is not yet capable of specific immune reaction. In the paragraph on the role of the age in the induction of tolerance I have given evidence suggesting that young animals, in which tolerance is generally the easiest to induce, already have the capacity to react against the inducing antigens by immune reaction. Moreover, evidence is presented there that immunological tolerance can be induced even in adult individuals. In this situation the question arises whether the induction of tolerance is not mediated through an immune reaction which as a result of antigen excess leads to its exhaustion and subsequent non-reactivity. This view has been put forward by ŠTERZL and TRNKA [1957] on the basis of their experiments with bacterial antigen. They found that an increase in its dose injected into newborn rabbits led to an earlier and stronger antibody response. However, when these animals were re-vaccinated, their antibody titres were much lower than in animals not injected with antigen at birth. This finding was surprising because a secondary response was to be expected.

Similar results were obtained by ŠTERZL [1966] with sheep erythrocytes in newborn rabbits and piglets. The response to injected erythrocytes was ascertained at the cellular level by determining antibody-forming cells using the method of localized haemolysis in gel. The highest dose of erythrocytes given after birth (2×10^{10} for rabbits and 2×10^{11} for piglets) provoked the strongest reaction in the young of both species. Upon reimmunization at the age of three weeks, however, the number of antibody-forming cells was lower in this group than in groups injected with lower doses at birth. In rabbits, the response in this group was even lower than in the group not injected with antigen at birth.

In the light of their results these authors proposed a hypothesis of the mechanism involved in immunological tolerance. They assume that a dual contact with antigen is necessary for the differentiation of immunologically competent cells into antibody-forming cells. Upon administration of a large dose of antigen this dual contact is accomplished in most of the immunologically competent cells and they are differentiated into antibody-forming cells of short life-span. These cells do not further proliferate and thus a much lower number of compatible cells is available on the second contact with antigen than on the first. When antigen is given in smaller doses the cells are activated, but antigen is lacking for their further differentiation. The activated cells proliferate and upon further supply of antigen form a basis for a more intense reaction – the secondary response.

If this hypothesis were true, then the phase of immune reaction would precede the phase of unresponsiveness in the induction of each state of tolerance. This hypothesis may be most easily refuted by the observation of the tolerant state not preceded by immune reaction. With regard to the large amount of antigen generally needed for the induction of tolerance it would be desirable to demonstrate the absence of immune reaction at the cellular level where the danger of masking with antigen excess may be more easily excluded than at the effector level. No work exists, to my knowledge, that would attempt to provide such evidence. For this reason I will cite some results from this laboratory; although they do not give conclusive evidence, they at least put forward data at variance with the above hypothesis.

Studies on the elimination of various doses of HSA from the circulation of chickens have shown that the immune elimination starts after massive doses of antigen (0.5 and especially 2.5 g/KBW) later than after the tens of milligramme quantities generally used for

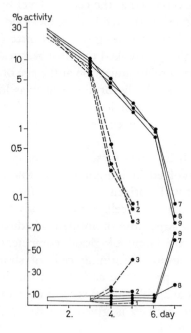

Fig. 4. Antigen and antigen-antibody complexes in the blood of chickens injected with different doses of HSA. - - - - - - - = 10 mg ^{131}I-HSA/KBW; ———— = 10 mg ^{131}I-HSA/KBW combined with 2.0 g HSA/KBW; x = days after antigen injection; y (left) = percentage of the original radioactivity in serum; y (right) = percentage of total radioactivity contained in antigen-antibody complexes.

immunization [Iványi et al., 1964b]. The shape of the elimination curve with a sudden onset of the immune elimination phase of antigen was at variance with the explanation that the delay in the onset of immune elimination might actually be a masking of antibody production by excess antigen present in the circulation. Another piece of evidence against this explanation was the finding that circulating antigen-antibody complexes demonstrable by the precipitation of ^{131}I-HSA with 50% saturated ammonium sulphate [Farr, 1958] appear even after large doses of antigen until the immune elimination commences (Fig. 4). Direct evidence on the delayed onset of antibody formation following large doses of HSA was provided by the study of cells forming antibodies against HSA by means of an indirect fluorescence technique [Černý et al., 1965]. Antibody-forming cells could be demonstrated in the spleen of two out of three chickens injected with 25 mg HSA/KBW as early as two days (48 h) after injection. In the spleen of animals injected with a 100 times higher dose (2.5 g/KBW) antibody-forming cells were detected in only one out of four animals as late as four days after injection (Table II).

Table II. Number of antibody-forming cells in spleens of chickens injected with HSA

Days after HSA injection	Dose of HSA injected	
	25 mg/KBW	2500 mg/KBW
2	>1[a, b], 1, 0	
3	3, 7, 15, 20	0, 0, 0, 0
4	11, 25, 30, 130	0, 0, 0, 3
5	13, 16, 90, 90	>1, >1, 2, 7
6	>1, 2, 2, 10	0, 9, 9, 14
7	0, >1, 1	2, 7, 12, 13

Anti-HSA forming cells were detected by immunofluorescence in imprints from the spleens.

[a] Number of antibody-forming cells in 20 mm² of the imprint. Each number represents the value determined in one animal.

[b] Antibody-forming cells were detected, but their frequency was less than 1 cell/20 mm² of the imprint.

After Černý et al. [1965].

The possibility has been excluded that a large amount of antigen may interfere with the detection of antibody-forming cells [ČERNÝ and IVÁNYI, 1966]; the animals were immunized with 1 mg HSA and after four days were inoculated with 2 g HSA. Four hours later, they were sacrificed. In this group the number of antibody-forming cells was not much lower than that in the group given only the immunizing dose of 1 mg HSA four days prior to examination (80 cells/area as compared with 100 cells/area). Similar results were obtained in the group of animals injected in the beginning of the experiment with 100 mg HSA instead of 1 mg. The spleen was examined on the 5th day. When these animals were injected with 2 g HSA on the 4th day, or with 2 g on the 3rd and 1 g HSA on the fourth day the number of antibody-forming cells was twice as large as that observed in the group injected only with 100 mg HSA (140 and 136 cells/area as compared with 70 cells/area). Later onset of antibody formation following large doses of antigen has also been confirmed by longer duration of the actinomycin-D sensitive phase of antibody-synthesis [SERCARZ et al., 1967].

A quantitative study of HSA elimination from the circulation of chickens revealed another interesting dependence [IVÁNYI and ČERNÝ, 1965]. With lower doses of antigen, the difference in the time of onset of immune elimination is small and the level of HSA in the circulation at the time of its onset increases linearly with increasing dose of antigen injected. On the other hand, with large doses of antigen, its immune elimination does not start until its concentration in the blood falls to approximately 0.1 mg/ml independently of the increase in antigen dose injected (Fig. 5). Just within the range of these doses the catabolic phase of antigen elimination was prolonged and the onset of immune elimination was delayed. The higher concentration of antigen in the circulation seems to inhibit in some way the onset of antibody formation.

In further experiments it has been demonstrated that no immune reactions are manifest as long as the chickens are injected repeatedly with high doses of HSA [ČERNÝ and IVÁNYI, 1966]. The series of injections of HSA was started with a dose of 2 g, and thereafter every 24 hours 1 g HSA was inoculated. In a group of 12 chickens so treated, 4 animals were sacrificed on the 4th, 7th and 12th day respectively. In 480 imprints made from their spleens (about 10^7 cells) not a single antibody-forming cell was detected.

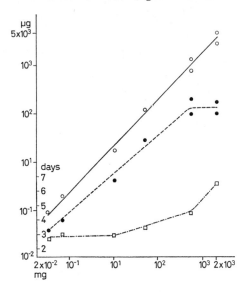

Fig. 5. Effect of HSA dose on its concentration in the blood on day of onset of immune elimination. ———— = antigen concentration on the 1st day after injection; ———— = antigen concentration on the day of onset of immune elimination; —·—·—·— = day of onset of immune elimination. Each circle represents the mean value of one experimental group. x = mg ^{131}I-HSA/KBW injected intravenously; y (left) = µg ^{131}I-HSA in 1 ml blood; y (right) = days after injection [after IvÁNYI and ČERNÝ, 1965].

These findings support the view that tolerance if induced by a sufficiently high dose of antigen may develop without a preceding immune phase. However, the inhibition of antibody formation by a high concentration of antigen cannot be considered as tolerance. As mentioned above, in this case a decrease in the concentration of antigen below a relatively high level results in the onset of immune reaction. Experiments in which a long-term maintenance of a high level of antigen prevented the onset of the immune reaction support the view that such an inhibition by excess antigen, if it lasts long enough, might go over to immunological tolerance. Data, in fact, are available that inhibition of antibody formation can be obtained by a similar series of injections of large doses of HSA in chickens [IvÁNYI *et al.*, 1964a]. Such data are, however, lacking for the group in which inhibition of antibody formation has been studied at the cellular level; hence the possibility of comparing both these experimental series is limited, as the reactions of different groups of chickens vary considerably. Moreover, inhibition of antibody formation obtained in the above experiments was only partial in young animals which were also used in the second experiment.

Another indirect but much more convincing piece of evidence supports the view that an immune reaction need not occur during induction of tolerance. Tolerance can be induced by some substances that are themselves unable to elicit an immune reaction. The first findings of this kind were made by DRESSER [1962b]. The BGG preparation he used in his experiments appeared to be a very poor antigen when injected in saline into mice. The preparation freed of all particulate matter by ultracentrifugation lost all its antigenicity, but it regained it when injected in adjuvant [DRESSER, 1961a]. The injection of centrifuged preparation without adjuvant did not immunize adult mice but rendered them tolerant of BGG [DRESSER, 1962b]. A similar inhibition was obtained in adult rabbits by the injection of hare γ-globulin, but not of BGG [DRESSER and GOWLAND, 1964].

Furthermore, it has been shown that tolerance can be induced with synthetic, multi-chain poly-DL-alanine. This polypeptide is not capable of eliciting an immune response, but antibodies against it are formed when it is bound to a protein carrier. Rabbits injected at birth with this polypeptide were found not to form antibodies against it upon challenge with polypeptide-carrier conjugate [SCHECHTER et al., 1964].

In the case of the Sulzberger-Chase phenomenon, the substances eliciting inhibition of immune reaction are also haptens; they are low-molecular-weight and very simple substances. It is possible to induce and test contact sensitivity by application of these haptens alone to the skin. In this case, these substances are bound to macromolecular components of the body of the tested animal and thus form a complete antigen. The same probably happens during the induction of unresponsiveness.

An attempt to induce tolerance to a simple hapten without a carrier was made by BOYDEN and SORKIN [1962]. Rabbits were injected at birth with sodium sulphanilate and challenged with sulphanil-HSA. After challenge all the treated rabbits produced antibody against the sulphanilic acid, in the same titre as control animals. It is questionable whether tolerance induced by hapten which would conjugate with the host's own substances might be detected after immunization with hapten on a heterologous carrier. Tolerance induced by a hapten on a heterologous carrier was found to inhibit the formation of antibody against the hapten on the carrier used for induction of tolerance as well as on an autologous one, but not on another heterologous carrier [WEIGLE, 1965].

Successful induction of tolerance to a simple chemical hapten was described by JONES and LESKOWITZ [1965] in guinea-pigs. They suppressed delayed hypersensitivity to arsanilic acid by the injection of both an antigenic substance such as arsanil-polytyrosine or arsanil-BSA and low-molecular-weight arsanil-tyrosine into newborn guinea-pigs. No inhibition occurred after arsanilic acid alone. The above substances can desensitize delayed hypersensitivity in immune guinea-pigs, but this kind of effect could hardly be manifest in these experiments, for the inhibition was also detectable here after the same dose of arsanil-tyrosine by the 8th week after birth, while the desensitization lasted only 5 days. The question remains open whether this hapten produces tolerance as a low-molecular-weight substance, or whether it becomes a complete antigen in the body. Doubts on this point are strengthened by the finding that some low-molecular-weight derivatives of tyrosine are capable of inducing both delayed hypersensitivity [LESKOWITZ et al., 1966] and formation of circulating antibodies [BOREK et al., 1965] when injected in complete Freund's adjuvant.

All the results I have outlined on the possibility of tolerance induction by means of substances unable themselves to induce immune response seem to provide very strong support for the view that the induction of tolerance is not mediated through an immune reaction. An objection may be raised that tolerance is induced after the administration of these substances through a different mechanism than after the administration of complete antigens. No experimental evidence is, however, available to lend support to the assumption of the existence of such a dual mechanism.

A very important finding relevant to this discussion was made by MITCHISON [1964]. He succeeded to induce tolerance to BSA in adult mice by repeated injections of not only high, but also low doses of antigen. The low doses capable to effect this inhibition are smaller than immunogenic ones. It is therefore possible with this antigen to induce tolerance at two levels of antigen dosage—high and low—which are separated by a zone of dosages inducing immunity.

It will have to be established, whether generally subimmunogenic doses of antigen can induce tolerance. If this were the case, this would substantially change the prospects for the use of tolerance in medicine.

However, the possibility is not excluded that this phenomenon is caused by the presence of two different forms of BSA in the preparation used: one aggregated and immunogenic and the other non-aggregated and lacking immunogenicity. This is suggested by the findings of FREI et al. [1965]. They succeeded in inducing tolerance to BSA in adult rabbits by injecting them with the serum of another rabbit previously injected with BSA. They assumed that the BSA in the serum was largely in the nonaggregated form and that the aggregated form had been cleared by the RES of the donor rabbit. Possibly in the low dose tolerance in mice, this immunogenic form of antigen is present in subimmunogenic quantities, while the non-immunogenic form of BSA is still present in quantities which can induce tolerance in the absence of immune reaction.

Regardless of the mechanism involved in low dose tolerance, it seems improbable that the initial phase of the induction of this type of tolerance would be an immune reaction.

On the basis of our experiments on the suppression of the immune reaction by large doses of antigen I assume that such doses are capable of inducing tolerance before an immune reaction takes place, or of preventing the development of an immune reaction up to the induction of complete tolerance. However, even a dose smaller than that needed for the suppression of an immune reaction by excess antigen, when given repeatedly, may obviously induce tolerance. Such doses of antigen initially elicit immunity in some cells of the lymphoid population. If the supply of antigen is continued, the immune reaction may be gradually suppressed and the resultant state is complete tolerance. In this context it is very important that immunological tolerance can be induced even in preimmunized animals. This question has been widely studied using pneumoccal polysaccharides and heterologous serum proteins. FELTON et al. [1955a] induced paralysis to pneumococcal polysaccharide in animals preimmunized against it. The amount of antigen needed was, however, much higher than that for non-immune mice. On the other hand, SISKIND and HOWARD [1966] failed to find that higher quantities of polysaccharide were needed for the induction of paralysis in immune mice; these appeared to be even more susceptible to it than non-immune animals.

DORNER and UHR [1964a, b] induced tolerance to BSA in about half the rabbits in which the immune reaction had previously been elicited and proved by immune elimination of antigen from the circulation. It is surprising that the dose used was relatively small: 200 mg BSA injected daily over 21 days. The animals were tested for tolerance by the elimination of antigen and serologically, and the immune reaction was not detectable by any of these tests in tolerant individuals. DRESSER [1965] was successful in producing strong inhibition of immune reaction in mice preimmunized with BGG in complete Freund's adjuvant. The doses of antigen needed were, however, much higher than those in non-immunized animals. He found further that the dose of antigen required for the induction increased as the intensity of immunity produced by preimmunization was stronger. On the other hand, X-irradiation increased the ability of antigen to induce tolerance. In the light of his experiments he concluded that circulating antibodies could hardly play an important role in the change of antigen dose inducing tolerance and that the reduced capacity to induce tolerance in preimmunized animals might have been due to intracellular antibodies.

An interesting system in which the immune reaction is suppressed, probably due to tolerance induction in the lymphoid cells of preimmunized animals, has been described by MARK and DIXON [1963]. Lymphoid cells from preimmunized mice were exposed *in vitro* to various concentrations of heterologous protein used for the immunization of donors, and then transferred to irradiated recipients. The reaction of cells exposed to large doses of antigen had a lower intensity than of those exposed to smaller doses. Under similar experimental conditions, however, MÄKELÄ and MITCHISON [1965b] observed stimulation after incubation of cells with high concentrations of antigen. When they transferred lymphoid cells from preimmunized animals to irradiated recipients and thereafter tested the immune reaction by the injection of various doses of antigen into the recipients, they also observed inhibition of antibody formation following large doses. The doses of antigen that had induced the immune response stimulated at the same time the proliferation of transferred lymphoid cells, as was revealed by the incorporation of a radioactively labelled analogue of thymidine. Large doses of antigen did not stimulate such proliferation.

A very interesting observation of the induction of immunological unresponsiveness in preimmunized mice has been made by CROWLE [1963]. He immunized mice with ovalbumin in complete Freund's adjuvant. Three weeks later the mice were desensitized by a series of antigen injections given daily for seven successive days. The reactivity of mice in both the immediate and delayed reaction to antigen fell markedly, but rapidly returned to normal in all animals when the course of desensitizing injections was terminated. While hypersensitivity of the delayed type persisted in most of the sensitized control animals throughout the observation period (4 months), it began to disappear rapidly and was retained in only a minor part of the desensitized animals after a transient return of reactivity. A similar, though not so obvious, course was noted with immediate hypersensitivity. Short-term desensitization was superseded by a permanent inhibition in this experiment.

The encounter of cells engaged in immune reactions, elicited by preimmunization and probably of those occurring during induction of tolerance, with antigen excess, may be associated with their irreversible damage. The morphology of cellular changes in the lymphoid organs in a similar experimental situation has been studied by CHUTNÁ and RYCHLÍKOVÁ [1966]. They tried to inhibit the immune reaction by massive doses of testicular antigen in saline in guinea-pigs, in which allergic aspermatogenesis was produced by the injection of testicular extract in complete Freund's adjuvant. The dose of 2 g testicular homogenate was injected twice, on the 10th and 13th day after immunization with the same antigen in complete Freund's adjuvant. At that time the lesions of spermatogenesis started to develop. The development of the lesions was stopped in animals given a massive injection of the homogenate and the state of spermatogenesis began to improve. In most animals treated in this way no immune reactions detectable serologically or by skin tests could be found. After the administration of massive doses of antigen the number of blast cells in the spleen and lymph nodes fell very rapidly to the values observed in non-immunized animals (1–2%). These values remained at the level of approximately 10% in animals immunized only with antigen in adjuvant (Fig. 6). On the other hand, the number of plasma cells in these organs increased immediately after massive doses of antigen, but fell later to the values similar to those observed in non-immune animals. However, many cells in the spleen and lymph nodes were considerably damaged after the injection of the homogenate in saline. As early as 24 h after the second injection of the large dose of antigen the cytological picture of these lymphoid organs was characterized by numerous damaged and disintegrating cells, some of which could still be identified mainly as plasmocytes. The extent of the damage was greater in the spleen than in the lymph nodes at first and the damaged cells disappeared more rapidly in the spleen (Fig. 7). The results of this experiment also suggest that not only desensitization but also a more permanent inhibition of the immune reaction has been achieved by antigen excess.

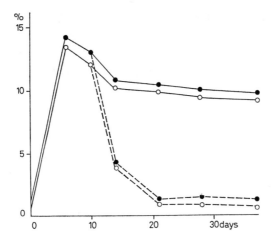

Fig. 6. Blast cells in lymph nodes and spleens of guinea-pigs injected with testicular extract. ———— = animals injected with extract in complete Freund's adjuvant only; – – – – – – = animals injected with extract in adjuvant and 10 and 13 days later with its massive dose in saline; ● = mean value of blast cells in lymph nodes; ○ = mean values of blast cells in spleen; x = days after injection of antigen in adjuvant; y = percentage of blast cells in the cell population of the lymph node [after Chutná and Rychlíková, 1966].

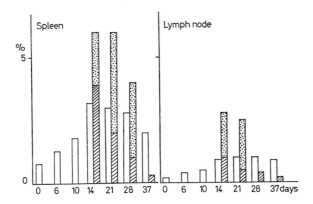

Fig. 7. Plasma cells in spleen and lymph nodes of guinea-pigs injected with testicular extract. ☐ = animals injected with extract in complete Freund's adjuvant only; ▤ = animals injected with extract in adjuvant and 10 and 13 days later with its massive dose in saline; ▦ = dead cells in the organs of animals of the preceding group. x = days after injection of antigen in adjuvant [after Chutná and Rychlíková, 1966].

A concomitant induction of tolerance and priming after the injection of *S. adelaide* flagellin into newborn rats, as observed by NOSSAL and AUSTIN [1966], is obviously another example of the situation in which the antigen inducing tolerance elicits at the same time an immune reaction. In this case, the induction of antibody formation is not directly involved, but the formation of immunological memory. The authors assume that the development of cells responsible for immunological memory proceeds along a different pathway from that of cells producing antibodies, and that these cells are not merely a transient stage in a series of cell transformations from immunologically competent cells up to antibody-forming cells. Even if this view were correct, the whole situation would resemble the development of antibody-forming cells during induction of tolerance. For example, also here repeated administration of small doses of antigen, at first evoking the occurrence of memory cells, leads later to their physical or functional elimination. NOSSAL and AUSTIN considered the possibility that this may take place as a result of the phase of transient sensitivity of these cells towards antigen.

A unique example of the induction of immunological tolerance in preimmunized animals is the re-induction of tolerance after it has disappeared. The re-induction is effected against immunity since the loss of tolerance is detected by the immune reaction coming in force after challenge. The phenomenon of re-induction of tolerance was observed by HAŠEK and PUZA [1962a, b] in experiments on embryonic parabionts between two species of ducks. In this combination, embryonic parabiosis gives rise to erythrocyte chimaerism which may be eliminated by the passive administration of antiserum. Tolerance to erythrocytes of the partner species detectable by non-immune elimination of ^{51}Cr-labelled erythrocytes from the circulation disappears within a few weeks after such abolition of chimaerism. However, massive transfusions of blood (3–4% body weight) from the partner of the other species given after tolerance was lost make tolerance to foreign erythrocytes re-appear. Transfusion of foreign blood in amounts corresponding to 6% body weight failed to induce tolerance in control ducks. A similar re-induction of tolerance has been performed by the above authors in Peking ducks rendered and maintained tolerant of erythrocytes of muscovy ducks by a course of blood injections, starting after hatching. After a course of injections had been stopped, tolerance disappeared, and this was also tested by elimination of erythrocytes. Transfusion of blood corresponding to 3–6% body weight was capable of restoring the state of tolerance to erythrocytes even in these animals.

The re-induction of tolerance in rabbits that had lost their unresponsiveness to heterologous serum proteins induced after birth was observed by HUMPHREY [1964 a]. The rabbits showing the signs of immune elimination of antigen were later retested with the same antigen. Of these, many showed no immune reaction after this new challenge. The dose of antigen used for test immunization was evidently sufficient to re-induce tolerance in them.

The most surprising feature in these findings was that although these animals reacted in an immune fashion against the previously tolerated antigens after tolerance had been lost, tolerance could be re-induced by a dose of antigen incapable of rendering non-immune individuals tolerant. This finding is a serious reminder that a weak immune reaction may easily escape detection during induction of tolerance and that it will be very difficult definitely to refute the view that immunological tolerance is induced through an immune reaction. Nevertheless, the results of the pertinent experiments and indirect evidence favour the hypothesis that the induction of tolerance is not effected in this way but through a different process.

(b) Immune Reaction after Disappearance of Tolerance

In addition to the period of tolerance induction during which the immune reaction may take place, the period after the loss of tolerance promises to furnish information on the nature of tolerance by analysing the immune reaction. The most important finding in this respect is that a spontaneous onset of immunity takes place after the termination of tolerance. This phenomenon has been observed so far only in mice and was described for the first time by TERRES and HUGHES [1959]. Mice given BSA at birth were unresponsive to it after challenge at the age of 6 weeks. Another group of these mice challenged at 12 weeks of age reacted by anaphylactic shock to this injection of BSA. Tolerance was no longer detectable, and they even formed antibody without an additional supply of antigen.

THORBECKE et al. [1961] found that immunological unresponsiveness induced in newborn mice by the injection of BGG later passed spontaneously into a phase of increased reactivity. They could not demonstrate circulating antibodies in these mice before challenge, but the subsequent immune reaction had the character of an anamnestic response. SERCARZ and COONS [1963] likewise observed a spontaneous onset of antibody formation in mice after a series of BSA injections starting at birth. Since injections of alum-precipitated BSA were included in this series, the spontaneity of this escape is not quite certain. COONS [1963], however, found a spontaneous onset of antibody formation in the group of mice given a series of ovalbumin injections from birth and not injected with alum-precipitated antigen.

In a further work SOREM and TERRES [1963] analysed this question in mice injected at birth with BSA. They found that the phase of unresponsiveness, the duration of which was lengthened as the amount of injected antigen increased, was followed by a phase during which the animals did not synthesize antibody but were primed to do so after challenge. The third phase was characterized by the production of antibody in the absence of challenge.

A spontaneous onset of an immune reaction after the previous phase of unresponsiveness in mice has also been described after the neonatal injection of pneumococcal polysaccharide [SISKIND et al., 1963]. No such phenomenon has been observed in any other animal species. So far as I know there is no work dealing directly with this question where spontaneous appearance of antibodies after the loss of unresponsiveness has been observed at different time intervals. Indirect evidence against the transition of tolerance into spontaneous antibody formation, or at least a state of increased reactivity, may be seen in the findings obtained in chickens whose immune response after the loss of tolerance to foreign erythrocytes and heterologous proteins was no stronger than in the controls. The significance of some of these observations is weakened by the fact that the animals were challenged during the observation period. However, this was avoided in the work in which we ourselves studied the nature of antibodies in chickens after the loss of tolerance to HSA [IVÁNYI and HRABA, 1964]. Tolerance was induced by a single injection of a large dose of antigen (50, 100 or 200 mg) given within 48 h of birth. Such a dose induced tolerance detectable at the age of 6–8 weeks [IVÁNYI and HRABA, 1963]. In this experiment challenge was postponed to the 12th week after hatching, when tolerance was presumed to be lost. This expectation was confirmed. Using three different methods (quantitative precipitation, passive haemagglutination and the Farr technique) the amount of antibody against HSA found in serum collected on the 7th day after immunization was the same in the groups of chickens injected at birth and in the control group. Individual sera were pooled because of their small variability within the groups; these pools were used to follow the course of the quantitative precipitation with ^{131}I HSA, to determine the sedimentation characteristics of HSA antibodies, their resistance to 2-ME, and finally, their avidity by means of the Farr technique using two different concentrations of antigen and determining the rate of dissociation. Not only was the amount of antibodies produced the same in all groups injected after hatching and in control groups, but also none of the methods used revealed any difference in the nature of antibodies between the different experimental groups.

Similar data on the nature of antibodies after termination of tolerance to BSA were obtained by DIETRICH and GREY [1964] in mice. They induced tolerance with a single injection of 20 mg BSA into newborn mice, and challenge with the same antigen in complete Freund's adjuvant was performed at the age of 10 weeks. Twenty-five days after challenge the antibody titre was lower in the tolerant group than in the control group, and the dissociation of antigen-antibody complexes was higher in neonatally injected mice than in the controls. However, the same titre and the same dissociation half-life were found in both groups 74 days after challenge. In this experiment, neither priming nor increase in immune reactivity towards the antigen used to induce tolerance were observed, but the difference in the quantity and quality of antibodies between both groups on the 25th day after challenge seemed to suggest that the neonatally injected group still showed some signs of tolerance. This might be the reason why no sensitization was observed in these mice similar to that observed after the termination of tolerance in the works earlier mentioned. The difference in the experimental results of different authors would, however, require a more detailed elucidation.

The spontaneous onset of an immune reaction after the termination of tolerance resembles the delayed onset of antibody formation after massive doses of HSA which has been observed in chickens [IVÁNYI et al., 1964 a; ČERNÝ et al., 1965]. The similarity between the two phenomena is still more accentuated as spontaneous onset of antibody formation during escape from tolerance seems to be due to the antigen persisting in the body. The results of DOWDEN and SERCARZ [1966] suggest that the primary change is loss of tolerance. Only then does the contact with antigen, either endogenous or newly administered one, initiate antibody formation. The difference may be seen in that the level of antigen in the circulation is relatively high at a time when antibody formation starts, following a large dose of antigen in chickens, while it must be very low in paralysis with heterologous proteins in mice. The question is whether only this form of antigen plays a decisive role in the given phenomena. It is likely that antigen in another localization, probably phagocytized, might have greater importance in mice because large doses of antigen in experiments on mice acted for a longer time than in the experiments with chickens. Even in chickens the antigen in the circulation may not be a proper form which may directly act on the inhibition of the immune reaction, but since the antigen is supplied from this pool to the critical site, there is a good correlation between its level in the circulation and the inhibition achieved. Furthermore, the possibility is not excluded that the reason for the difference in the development of an immune reaction after the loss of tolerance between various species should be looked for in the different fate of antigen. Nevertheless, a considerable difference seems to exist between the antigenic requirements during unresponsiveness to heterologous proteins in rabbits on the one hand, and in mice and perhaps in chickens on the other. In rabbits tolerance may clearly persist even if minimal amounts of antigen remain in the organism, whereas much larger quantities must be present in the other two species. This difference raises the question whether in both cases the inhibition is due to the same mechanism. The central failure of the mechanism of immune reaction seems to be involved in both cases, but it is likely (and I think very probable) that several mechanisms might be operative.

(c) Abolition of Tolerance

The possibility of inducing autoimmune reactions by immunization with autologous or homologous material in complete Freund's adjuvant raises the question of whether or not immunization with a tolerated antigen in complete Freund's adjuvant leads to the abolition of tolerance. In the case of complete tolerance to heterologous proteins in rabbits, this method of immunization did not induce antibody formation [SMITH, 1961; WEIGLE, 1962]. Neither did the use of specific antigen-antibody complexes incorporated in complete Freund's adjuvant result in the abolition of tolerance [CHUTNÁ and HRABA, 1962; WEIGLE, 1962]. SMITH [1961] observed that such immunization at the end of the tolerance phase may shorten its duration to some extent. It is, however, possible that intensive immunization does not alter its duration but is capable of eliciting detectable antibody formation at an earlier date. We observed this in chickens in which partial tolerance to HSA had been induced by its administration after hatching [IVÁNYI and HRABA, 1963]. More chickens produced precipitins and in comparison with the controls in relatively larger amounts after an intense challenge with 200 mg HSA/KBW than after a dose of 40 mg/KBW.

The possibility is not excluded that immunization with a tolerated antigen in complete Freund's adjuvant, though not capable of abolishing tolerance immediately, has some effect and may shorten its duration. The action of complete Freund's adjuvant at the end of the period of tolerance could not then be reduced to a more intensive immunizing action. I am not aware of any observation that might help in solving this question.

It is necessary to mention the opposite results of NEEPER and SEASTOWNE [1963], who succeeded in abolishing paralysis to type I pneumococcal polysaccharide by immunization with, or after injection of, incomplete Freund's adjuvant. It is not clear whether the cause is to be sought in a relatively weak state of tolerance or elsewhere.

With the Sulzberger-Chase phenomenon it is also possible to induce skin sensitivity to the hapten used in non-reactive animals when they are sensitized by the combined method [CHASE, 1963; BATTISTO and CHASE, 1963]. This method [CHASE, 1954] consists in injecting the tested animals first with hapten conjugated to guinea-pig erythrocyte stromata incorporated in complete Freund's adjuvant. Thereafter the hapten solution is repeatedly applied to the skin of the animals. This method of sensitization is very effective; the reaction it induces in unresponsive guinea-pigs, however, is 50–100 times weaker than the reaction in the controls, and this difference seems to be permanent. It is not clear whether the use of adjuvant or some other factor might be responsible for the break down of tolerance, or whether this type of challenge reveals an incomplete state of unresponsiveness. The question of the effect of Freund's adjuvant on tolerance should be concluded by assuming that this effect is far from being so dramatic as in inducing experimental autoimmune syndromes.

Sublethal irradiation, which represents a profound intervention into the lymphoid tissue, could be expected to influence the state of tolerance. In young animals an intense cell proliferation is probably the important factor in a more rapid loss of tolerance and this suggests that irradiation may lead in a similar way to breakdown of tolerance. Attempts made by DENHARDT and OWEN [1960] failed to abolish tolerance of BSA in rabbits when exposed to whole-body irradiation of 300 r. On the other hand, in rats rendered tolerant by a series of

injections of mouse erythrocytes, or of BSA, starting after birth, irradiation with 550–600 r generally led to breakdown of tolerance and
to immune reaction of the same intensity as in the control group
[Mäkelä and Nossal, 1962]. Sublethal irradiation also broke down
transplantation tolerance induced by neonatal injections in mice
[Fefer and Nossal, 1962; Nossal et al., 1962].

On the other hand, immunization with antigens cross-reacting with
the tolerated antigen appeared to be a very effective tool in abolishing
tolerance. This finding is very important because it has been obtained
with such a stable state of tolerance as the unresponsiveness to heterologous proteins in rabbits. This phenomenon was observed for the
first time by Cinader and Dubert [1955, 1956] in rabbits tolerant of
HSA. Most of the tolerant animals did not form antibodies against
hapten or against the carrier protein when immunized with sulphanil-
HSA, but some of them formed antibodies reacting not only with sulphanil-HSA but also with native HSA.

After immunization of BSA-tolerant rabbits with other heterologous
serum albumins cross-reacting with the tolerated antigen Weigle
[1961] obtained antibody formation against both heterologous and
tolerated albumin. In this case, tolerance could be abolished more
readily by more distant and less cross-reacting antigens than by more
closely related ones. The tolerated antigen modified by binding of
chemical haptens was also capable of inducing the abolition of tolerance
[Weigle, 1962]. These results were at variance with the findings of
Boyden and Sorkin [1962]. They failed to find antibody formation
against the hapten and carrier protein when using sulphanil-HSA for
immunization of rabbits made tolerant of HSA by the administration
of antigen at an early age. When normal rabbits were immunized with
sulphanilic acid bound to rabbit serum albumin, the immunized animals produced antibody against the hapten. In addition to the difference between the results of the above authors, these findings seemed
to be at variance with the view that non-reactivity to indigenous components is effected through the same mechanism as tolerance to foreign
substances. Nachtigal and Feldman [1964] studied this question in
rabbits rendered tolerant to HSA following X-irradiation in adult life.

They found that the tolerant rabbits at first formed no antibody, but then did so against the hapten following immunization with its conjugate with both their own and the tolerated protein. These antibodies were directed partly against the hapten itself and partly against the determinant including hapten and a portion of the carrier. However, they did not react with the carrier alone. Unresponsiveness against their own serum albumin appeared to be more stable than against the tolerated HSA because, upon further immunization, the tolerant rabbits began to form antibody even against HSA. At first directed against determinants other than those against which normal rabbits do react, but when the tolerant rabbits were not treated for 75 days and then re-challenged with native HSA, the antibodies produced were identical to those formed by normal rabbits. The breakdown of non-reactivity to rabbit serum albumin following immunization with its sulphanil conjugate has never been observed. A possible reason may be the presence of rabbit serum albumin in the body during immunization. When immunization of tolerant rabbits with sulphanil-HSA was performed with a concomitant injection of native HSA, it was impossible to abolish tolerance. A similar observation was reported by WEIGLE [1964 b].

Apart from discovering the possibility of abolishing tolerance with a cross-reactive antigen, these works brought forward information on the change of antigenicity due to tolerance. It appeared that the binding of hapten to the tolerated carrier did not lead at first to a reaction against it [BOYDEN and SORKIN, 1962; NACHTIGAL and FELDMAN, 1964]. Likewise, immunization of BSA-tolerant rabbits with an antigenically similar substance – sheep serum albumin – resulted neither in the abolition of tolerance to BSA nor in the formation of antibodies against sheep albumin [WEIGLE, 1961]. Similarly, rabbits tolerant of HGG of definite allotype did not form antibody against HGG of another allotype [WEIGLE and FUDENBERG, 1966]. Since a major part of the determinants of the antigen used is tolerated, the possibility of an immunogenetic action of its non-tolerated determinants is impaired. Thus the given substance becomes a very poor antigen. One must therefore be very cautious in coming to the conclusion that the absence of an immune reaction to the antigen used to induce tolerance may mean tolerance to all its antigenic determinants.

Of interest are the findings on the specificity of antibody produced during the abolition of tolerance. It has been shown by LINSCOTT and WEIGLE [1965] that antibodies against arsanil-sulphanil-BSA in rabbits, in which tolerance to BSA had been abolished by this substance, had a higher binding affinity to the hapten determinants than to determinants of the native protein carrier, compared to the controls.

Yoshimura and Cinader [1966] observed an interesting relationship between determinants evoking antibody formation and determinants to which the antibodies produced are bound. In contrast to the above results, after the termination of tolerance to HSA with oxazolonated HSA antibodies directed against the carrier are better adapted to the determinants of native than to those of the modified protein.

4. Specificity of Tolerance

The characteristics of immunological tolerance as a central inhibition specific for the inducing antigen is an important feature distinguishing it from other types of central inhibition. These are, for example, the inhibition states induced by X-irradiation, or drugs, where a central but general inhibition of immunological reactivity is involved. A certain non-specificity of immunological tolerance has been touched upon in the previous paragraph, i. e. reduction of the immunogenicity of non-tolerated determinants on an otherwise tolerated antigen.

In this chapter the relationship between specificity of immunological tolerance and specificity of the immune reaction will be considered, or more precisely, whether the cross-reactivity as observed in immune reactions might take effect in a corresponding way in immunological tolerance.

The specificity of tolerance has been postulated on the basis of observations with transplantation tolerance where it appeared to be limited to the donor used for its induction [Anderson et al., 1951; Billingham et al., 1952, 1953, 1956a; Hašek, 1954]. A further study, however, showed that this specificity need not be complete [Terasaki et al., 1958; Billingham and Brent, 1959]. It was not clear whether the manifestation of unspecific suppression was due to antigenic similarity, or certain non-specificity of immunological tolerance was involved here. In interspecies relationships, the findings seem to suggest the latter possibility. In interspecies parabionts, the tolerance to erythrocytes and grafts of other individuals of the partner's species is mostly the same as to the cells of the parabiotic partner. Since this tolerance is generally only partial, this situation does not help in resolving this question. With tolerance to foreign cells, a non-specificity has been observed which is difficult to explain by antigenic overlapping or by reduction of antigenicity as a result of sharing in common the tolerated determinants. It has been shown that in embryonic parabionts between turkey and chicken the survival of allogeneic grafts is markedly prolonged even in animals with relatively poor tolerance to skin grafts from individuals of the partner species [HAŠEK et al., 1959, 1960; HAŠEK and HORT, 1960] (Fig. 8). The rejection of xenogeneic grafts from the species other than that to the cells of which tolerance had been induced proceeded at the same rate as in control animals. A similar situation was observed in interspecific parabionts between the domestic and the muscovy duck [HAŠEK, 1962; HAŠEK and HORT, 1962; HAŠEK et al., 1963]. It seems unlikely that this reduction of reactivity is due to some antigens of xenogeneic cells to which tolerance has been induced. It seems that tolerance to a stronger antigen suppresses the reactivity towards a weaker, probably not cross-reacting antigen, but does not affect the reactivity to other strong antigens. On the other hand, it is possible that the reactivity to strong antigens only *seems* to be unchanged. The reduction of immunological reactivity to all antigens can be involved. This might occur if interspecific chimaerism, at least temporarily existing in such parabionts, showed adverse effects on the development of their immunological reactivity. The possibility cannot be excluded that chimaerism persists for a long time in the lymphoid tissues although complete tolerance to the partner's antigens has not been induced

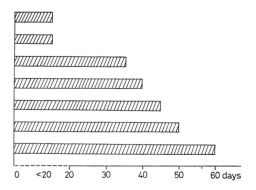

Fig. 8. Survival of allogeneic grafts in chicken parabionts with turkeys. Each bar represents survival of the graft in one parabiont. Survival of allogeneic grafts in normal animals and of xenogeneic grafts in both parabionts and controls was less than 20 days. x = days after transplantation [after HAŠEK et al., 1960].

or has been lost. In such cases, a graft-versus-host reaction may take place, and possibly *vice versa*, which may lead to an over-all damage to the host lymphoid tissues and to reduction of its immunological reactivity, more easily detectable when tested with a weak rather than a strong antigen.

With our material it was impossible to decide between these possibilities, but later findings suggested that the 'non-specificity of tolerance' was really involved. ZEISS [1966] succeeded in demonstrating in inbred strains of rats that the observed lack of specificity of transplantation tolerance was due neither to an antigenic overlapping with the donor whose cells had been used for the induction of tolerance nor to runt disease.

Systems using defined antigens are more suitable for the study of the specificity of tolerance. Evidence for the specificity of these phenomena has been given in the respective paragraphs. The findings showing non-specific tolerance and determining the limits of the specificity of tolerance in these systems will now be considered. The experiments of HANAN and OYAMA [1954], who induced tolerance to BSA in rabbits at an early age, revealed that the tolerant rabbits gave a significantly lower response to ovalbumin. However, SMITH and BRIDGES [1958] did not confirm this finding on their material. A similar non-specific non-reactivity was observed by HIRATA and SCHECHTMAN [1960]. Chickens rendered tolerant by the injection of HGG before hatching also showed significantly lower antibody production against BSA after challenge on the 45th day after hatching. Upon further challenge on the 100th day no decrease in antibody formation against HGG and BSA was detectable. Specific and 'non-specific' suppression disappeared in them simultaneously.

A similar observation was made by AUSTIN and NOSSAL [1966]. Rats made tolerant of antigen fg by a series of injections of monomeric flagellin responded normally to a number of unrelated antigens, but displayed a decreased or fully suppressed reaction to another two H-antigens of Salmonella (especially towards i, less towards d antigen). The tolerant animals reacted normally against flagellin of *Proteus vulgaris*. It could not be demonstrated that i and d antigens cross-reacted with the antigen used to induce tolerance. Further results obtained by these authors are of interest in the determination of the relationship between fg and i antigen. When both these antigens are injected simultaneously they do not influence antibody formation. However, if one of them is injected before the other, the immune reaction is reduced towards the antigen used as the second. To explain these phenomena the authors put forward the hypothesis that the immunologically competent cells from which the cells reacting against these antigens originate, are identical. Thus the pool of cells from which cells reacting with these antigens originate may be reduced or exhausted as a result of the induction of tolerance or of immune reaction to one of the antigens.

The data available permit some conclusions to be drawn regarding the size of the antigenic determinants involved in the states of tolerance. Such data were obtained during study of tolerance to low-molecular-weight chemical haptens. It has been shown by CINADER and PEARCE [1958] that rabbits injected at birth with a conjugate of sulphanilic acid with ribonuclease or rabbit serum formed antibodies against sulphanilic acid following immunization with sulphanil-HSA, whereas rabbits rendered tolerant by the injection of sulphanil-HSA failed to form them against both the hapten and the carrier. It appeared that tolerance could be induced only to a hapten bound to a certain carrier. When a hapten on a different carrier was used for testing, antibodies were formed against both carrier and hapten. WEIGLE [1965 a] induced tolerance to picrylated BSA in rabbits at birth. When these animals were immunized with another protein to which the picryl group was bound, they formed antibodies against this hapten as normal animals. No antibody formation against hapten was noted when picrylated rabbit serum albumin was used for immunization. Hence non-reactivity to both the tolerated carrier and its own protein may have a similar basis. Another of WEIGLE's findings that rabbits tolerant of picryl-BSA lost tolerance after immunization with sulphanil-BSA is of much interest for understanding the specificity of tolerance. Immunization of these rabbits with DNP-BSA did not lead to loss of tolerance to the carrier nor to antibody formation against the antigen used. The picryl and DNP group are similar serologically while the sulphanilic group is not. The difference between picryl-BSA and DNP-BSA is evidently not sufficient to lead to the abolition of tolerance or to immune reaction against the DNP group in the tolerant animals.

These results suggest that the part of the antigenic surface which is recognized during tolerance is greater than the antigenic determinant reacting with circulating antibody. In this respect the recognition in tolerance would be similar to that in secondary response and delayed hypersensitivity [MITCHISON, 1966]. The data available are, however, not sufficient for us to conclude that the size of the determinant is similar in all these cases and even that recognition is effected through the same mechanism in these instances. If non-specificity of tolerance to antigens which do not cross-react is due to low specificity of the antigen recognition, then it is probably different from the mechanism of recognition involved in the two immune manifestations mentioned. However, the mechanisms responsible for different manifestations of 'non-specificity' of tolerance may be different.

It is not clear how the above manifestations of 'non-specificity' of tolerance are associated with the suppression of an immune reaction to unrelated antigen during induction of immunological paralysis to heterologous serum proteins [LIACOPOULOS et al., 1962, 1963; LIACO-POULOS, 1961, 1965; LIACOPOULOS and NEVEU, 1964]. These authors produced paralysis to BSA in adult guinea-pigs by a series of injections given daily for 15-20 days. At different intervals after the commencement of this injection series the animals were inoculated with the immunizing dose of another antigen in alum-precipitated form. When the sensitizing injection was given together with the first injection of the paralysing antigen, the immune reaction was the same in paralysed and control animals. The intensity of the immune reaction and the number of sensitized animals decreased up to complete suppression of sensitization as the interval between the commencement of the paralysing injections and the sensitizing injections was extended. After termination of the series of the paralysing injections the reactivity to sensitizing injections of another antigen returned to its normal level very rapidly, but non-reactivity induced to such an antigen during induction of paralysis persisted even after the cessation of the paralysing treatment. Thus the guinea-pigs paralysed with BSA, which were made non-reactive during induction of paralysis by the injection of rabbit γ-globulin, did not react over two months after the first injection to a challenge with rabbit γ-globulin. Only after an additional challenge made a month later did they respond by a typical primary reaction. The sensitization induced against unrelated antigen prior to the induction of paralysis is not inhibited and the animals tested after the induction of paralysis with antigen used for sensitization react by secondary response. In this way, complete suppression of delayed hypersensitivity can be achieved, though not so easily as the suppression of circulating antibody [NEVEU et al., 1963]. The possible cause of this difference may be that complete Freund's adjuvant is used for challenge in these experiments and this is a strong immunizing stimulus capable of revealing even low reactivity.

Repeated massive injections of rabbit γ-globulin in mice led to a decrease in the capacity of their lymphoid cells to react against antigens of the irradiated recipient to which they were transfered, and facilitated the induction of tolerance to donor skin grafts in the recipient [LIACO-POULOS and STIFFEL, 1963; LIACOPOULOS and GOODE, 1964]. The induction of paralysis with heterologous proteins also produced some prolongation in the survival of skin allografts in rabbits [HALPERN et al., 1963].

The above authors assume that there is an antigenic competition leading to a decrease of the immune reaction, as has often been observed during simultaneous or subsequent immunization with different antigens [ADLER, 1964]. Of particular interest in this respect are the findings of NEVEU [1964] who found that the incorporation of two antigens in complete Freund's adjuvant led to a substantially greater inhibition of the immune reaction than a concomitant administration of antigens into different sites. Also autologous proteins incorporated with antigen in the mixture used showed the inhibitory effects, though less pronounced than foreign substances. The inhibition is evidently more intense when the two substances act simultaneously on the same part of the lymphoid tissue. The findings reported lend support to the view that immune reactions against different antigens compete for the same cells. It is, however, questionable whether immunologically competent cells or cells performing some non-specific operation with the given antigen are involved. Other explanations are also possible, so that these results cannot solve this problem.

It is not clear whether the competition of antigens during tolerance and immunity is effected through the same mechanism. Doubts on this point are well justified. The findings reported above speak for a non-specific decrease in immunological reactivity during induction of paralysis as the doses of antigen used are considerable and must be a great physiological stress for the organism.

This phenomenon must be further investigated in detail because of its theoretical significance and the possible practical applications, especially in tissue transplantations.

5. Reactions to the Tolerated Antigen

(a) The Fate of Tolerated Antigen in the Organism

Evidence reported in the previous chapters suggests that immunological tolerance as a state of immunological suppression due to specific central failure of the immune mechanism does really exist, and that this immunological suppression may be complete and may involve all types of immune reaction. In all probability, its induction is not mediated through the exhaustion of immune reaction. In this situation the question arises as to what reactions may take place upon introduction of the tolerated antigen: whether they are similar to those reactions preceding antibody formation during an immune reaction, or whether they may be different.

The original hypothesis of Burnet and Fenner [1949] postulated that tolerance is a mechanism through which non-reactivity to the organism's own components is effected. The antigen to which tolerance has been induced experimentally should also be recognized and dealt with as 'self' by the organism. It cannot be said that our information about the fate of the own worn-out components is satisfactory, but if we adopt this view as a working hypothesis, we can expect that the fate of antigen in tolerant animals will be different from that in animals capable of an immune reaction to the given antigen.

The most widely used method in the study of tolerance to heterologous serum proteins is the elimination of antigen from the circulation. Complete tolerance is manifested by the same rate of elimination throughout the whole period and identical with the rate during the catabolic phase in normal animals. The immune phase with an accelerated elimination of antigen present in control animals after the catabolic phase does not occur in tolerant animals. The follow-up of elimination of antigen is virtually a method demonstrating the immune reaction and informing us about that phase of disposal of antigen, which is of minor interest. The rate of non-immune elimination being the same for tolerant and normal animals before the onset of antibody formation suggests that the antigen is cleared from the circulation in the same way. This view is supported by the findings of Crampton and his associates [1959]. They induced tolerance to strongly iodinated heterologous proteins in rabbits by a series of injections which started at birth. The fate of the antigen labelled with radioactive iodine was followed in experimental and control animals at the age of 4–6 months. The antigen disappeared from serum within 24 h. Its distribution in the organs and the subcellular fractions followed 2 min to 24 h after injection was the same in tolerant and control animals which did not yet form antibody.

Similar results were obtained by Garvey et al. [1960]. Tolerance was induced in newborn rabbits by the injection of 20 mg sulphanil-

BSA labelled with radioactive sulphur. These animals and their siblings not injected at birth were challenged when 2 months old. Injected animals were tolerant of this antigen and did not form any antibody against it, whereas all control animals did so. Three weeks after challenge, the organ and subcellular distribution of antigen was followed. Again no substantial difference was found between the two groups of animals, though the control animals reacted by antibody formation.

The results on the localization of tolerated antigen obtained by Nossal and his colleagues [Nossal and Ada, 1964; Ada et al., 1965b] were surprising. They used in their experiments the flagellar protein of S. adelaide, which is highly immunogenic, so that really minimal amounts of antigen can be used for immunization. It is possible to induce a state of tolerance in rats with no formation of circulating antibody by relatively small amounts of antigen given in a series of injections starting at birth. It was unexpected that in tolerant animals the antigen was localized in the regional lymph nodes as in pre-immunized animals. This is of particular interest because this mode of localization is due to circulating antibodies [Nossal et al., 1965]. In this case, tolerance does not appear to be complete; this may be due either to the serological method incapable of detecting small amounts of antibody which were sufficient to produce an immune localization, or to the formation of opsonizing antibodies to this antigen which was not suppressed or only partially suppressed in spite of complete inhibition of serologically detectable antibodies. The possibility remains open that an immune reaction to the antigenic admixture of the flagellin preparation is in fact involved.

The assumption that in tolerant animals the fate of antigen would be different from that in normal animals has not yet been supported by any experimental results. It must be admitted that few suitable detection systems are available and the observations carried out so far are relatively scanty.

(b) Cell Reactions to the Tolerated Antigen

The introduction of antigen at first elicits the proliferation of lymphoid tissues and the increase in number of large pyroninophilic or blast cells and then the production of antibodies. The course of this reaction after the introduction of a tolerated antigen is very important for the understanding of the mechanism both of tolerance and of specific immune reactions. Turk and Stone [1963] made guinea-pigs non-reactive to dinitrochlorbenzene by an intravenous injection and found that the number of blast cells in the imprints made from their regional lymph nodes did not increase after the cutaneous application of the hapten. On the other hand, mice with neonatally induced tolerance to HSA were shown by Mathé et al. [1963] to contain after challenge in the regional lymph nodes the same number of hyperbasophilic cells as the controls. The results with transplantation tolerance obtained by Argyris [1963] also suggested that the proliferative reaction to a tolerated antigen took place in the lymphoid tissues of tolerant animals.

We studied this question in rabbits rendered tolerant to HSA at birth [Zaleski et al., 1966]. Cytological analyses were performed in smears of cell suspensions prepared from the regional lymph nodes [Zaleski et al., 1964]. In comparison with the results of the authors mentioned above, the data obtained by this method had the advantage that a representative sample of the cell population of a given node could be studied quantitatively. A relatively large dose of antigen (200 mg) was needed to elicit a sufficiently intensive blastic reaction in the regional lymph nodes of normal animals. The cytological picture was studied at different time intervals after challenge. In control animals, the percentage of blast cells reached its maximum by the 7th day and their number decreased by the 10th day. In tolerant animals, a slight, though significant, increase in the number of blast cells was observed on the 5th day after challenge, and on the 7th day their values did not differ from the initial ones. In control animals the number of plasma cells rose more markedly than that of blast cells, whereas in tolerant animals it did not change significantly (Fig. 9).

This result seems to suggest that in tolerant animals the blastic reaction is completely suppressed, or at least considerably reduced. It is questionable whether a small increase in the number of blast cells as observed in tolerant animals is a reaction to the tolerated antigen or to other antigenic components in the HSA preparation used. On the basis of the electrophoretic determination it was estimated that about 4 mg of other proteins are present in 200 mg of the HSA preparation used. The preliminary experiments carried out to determine a suitable immunizing dose seem to indicate that this amount may be sufficient for the induction of a weak blastic reaction. The possibility cannot, however, be excluded that the reaction might have been directed against the tolerated antigen.

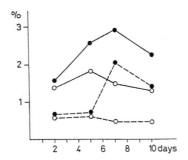

Fig. 9. Blast cells and plasmocytes in lymph nodes draining the injection site of HSA in rabbits. Challenge dose was 200 mg HSA per rabbit subcutaneously. ———— = mean value of blast cells; ——————— = mean value of plasmocytes; ● = mean value of the tolerant group; ○ = mean value of the control group; x = days after challenge; y = percentage of the respective cell type in lymph node cell population [after ZALESKI *et al.*, 1966].

The conclusion that a tolerated antigen does not lead to the proliferative reaction in the lymphoid tissues is in agreement with the finding of DUTTON [1964]. He showed that exposure of lymphoid cells from preimmunized donors to the antigen used for immunization led to a proliferative reaction; this was measured by the rate of incorporation of radioactive thymidine into the cells. When the cell suspension from tolerant, previously challenged animals was exposed to the tolerated antigen, no increased incorporation of thymidine was observed. COHEN and THORBECKE [1964] obtained interesting data. They suppressed the cell reaction to alum-precipitated BSA in the regional lymph nodes of very young rabbits by an intraperitoneal injection of dissolved BSA which in this situation induces tolerance. From this it seems probable that the blastic reaction is also absent during the induction of tolerance. Thus it appears that the proliferative and blastic reactions of the lymphoid tissues belong to specific immune reactions which are suppressed in immunological tolerance.

(c) Cells Mediating the Induction of Tolerance

Our knowledge of this aspect of the subject is very limited and this question is largely a matter of conjecture. I will therefore concentrate on two lines of investigation that seem of special relevance to the subject. The first are findings on the role of the thymus in tolerance. It has been shown that thymectomy in mice made tolerant to BGG at birth slows down but does not suppress escape from tolerance [Claman and Talmage, 1963]. Similar results were obtained by Taylor [1964] with tolerance to BGG and BSA. The thymus plays an important role in the recovery of immunological capacity of adult animals after whole-body irradiation or other depletion of the lymphoid system, and, as it seems, in the recovery from the specific suppression of the immune reaction in tolerance. However, the relationship between the thymus and tolerance may be more direct. Burnet's hypothesis [1962] that the thymus is an organ in which the elimination of reactivity to the own antigens of the organism takes place and the findings in autoimmune diseases supporting it [Burnet and Holmes, 1962; Arnason et al., 1962; Vojtíšková and Pokorná, 1964] instigated experiments trying to verify whether this organ also plays a similar role in the induction of tolerance to foreign antigens. Vojtíšková and Lengerová [1965] checked this hypothesis when inducing transplantation tolerance to a weak histocompatibility antigen. Foreign cells were allowed to enter the thymus either by direct injection, or after irradiation of the recipient whereby the functional barrier interfering with their entry into the thymus was removed. With these methods it was possible to induce tolerance to the cells used. The role of the thymus in the induction of tolerance was further confirmed [Vojtíšková and Lengerová, 1966] by transfer of the thymus from tolerant animals and especially from a hybrid between the donor and recipient strain to a lethally irradiated recipient protected by foetal liver cells of the same strain. The transfer of both organs, but particularly of the hybrid's thymus, can lead to the induction of permanent tolerance to skin grafts. Failure to obtain a similar effect by splenectomy and transplantation of spleen and lymph nodes indicates that the presence of antigen in the thymus is of decisive importance.

In rats, it has also been possible to transfer tolerance to BGG by the thymus from tolerant animals into irradiated thymectomized recipients [Isaković et al., 1965]. A similar effect was produced by transfer of thymus from normal animals injected with a large dose of BGG shortly before transfer [Smith et al., 1966] and the injection of antigen into the thymus of irradiated animals [Staples et al., 1966]. Toulette and Waksman [1966] succeeded in transferring transplantation tolerance by the thymus or by the injection of thymus cells from tolerant animals. On the other hand, Argyris [1966] transferred or induced transplantation tolerance in irradiated mice with spleen cells rather than thymus cells. The cause of the difference in these results is to be sought in the difference between the strain combinations used and in the experimental design.

Thus it appears that the thymus plays an important part in the induction and maintenance of tolerance, though it is not certain whether this part is indispensable. Some doubts on the necessity of the thymus in the induction of tolerance were cast by the finding of FOLLET et al. [1966] on the induction of the Sulzberger-Chase phenomenon by hapten bound to erythrocyte stromata; this was successful even in thymectomized animals. The action of the thymus in this respect may manifest itself by different mechanisms. I have in mind the prolongation of tolerance by thymectomy on the one hand, and transfer of tolerance by the thymus from tolerant animals on the other.

A second, very hopeful approach to the identification of cells engaged in tolerance is to prevent its induction by transfer of cells from normal animals into individuals in which tolerance is being induced. COHEN and THORBECKE [1963] prevented the induction of tolerance to BSA in newborn mice by transferring into them normal thymus and spleen cells on the first day after birth. FRIEDMAN [1964, 1965 c] was successful in preventing the induction of unresponsiveness to Shigella antigens in newborn mice by transfer of lymphoid cells from another donor simultaneously with the antigen or shortly after its injection. Cells from both newborn and adult animals, either normal or immune, were effective. Cells from animals rendered tolerant by a neonatal injection of antigen were also capable, after transfer of preventing the occurrence of tolerance in the recipient. Lymph node cells and spleen cells were approximately equally effective in preventing the occurrence of tolerance, thymus cells were less effective, peritoneal exudate cells still less effective, and bone marrow and buffy-coat cells ineffective.

This phenomenon was explained as being due to a shift in the proportion between the number of immunologically competent cells and the amount of antigen. Immunity or tolerance is presumed to occur to an extent which depends on the quantity of antigen per immunocompetent cell, not on the concentration in the organism. In addition to the difference in inducibility of tolerance between young and immunologically mature animals, this hypothesis satisfactorily explains the finding that tolerance can be maintained with very small doses of antigen, and that re-induction of tolerance, in spite of the existing immune reaction, may be achieved by the amount of antigen which is immunogenic for normal animals. Contrary to this idea is only the finding that the induction of tolerance can be prevented even by transfer of lymphoid cells from tolerant animals [FRIEDMAN, 1965c]. It is, however, difficult to imagine the mechanism which would depend upon the proportion between the number of immunologically competent cells and the amount of antigen in the whole body. It would be more feasible to assume that the mode of reaction of immunologically competent cells is determined by the concentration of antigen, either in their own environment or in a depot deciding their reaction. The hypothesis mentioned above has the advantage that it can be experimentally verified and thus from its being confirmed or refuted further data on the nature of immunological tolerance may be obtained.

The induction of tolerance to heterologous proteins injected into newborn rabbits could also be prevented by transfer of macrophages from adult donors [MARTIN, 1966].

The question is whether the inhibition of tolerance induction is effected through the same mechanism in all these experiments. This possibility is not excluded. It has been shown by CHOU et al. [1966] that the dose of antigen capable of eliciting tolerance in some newborn rabbits and not resulting in antibody formation in any of them gave rise to antibodies in newborns when administered bound to cells of a normal adult donor. This effect was displayed by cells from the lymph nodes, thymus and peritoneal exudate. The change in the immune reaction is evidently due to the different form of antigen introduced into newborn animals. Similarly, the administration of heterologous serum proteins in the form of a precipitate [CHUTNÁ and HRABA, 1962] or in complete Freund's adjuvant [PARAF et al., 1963] does not induce tolerance in newborn rabbits, but results in an immune reaction. Similar findings were made in monkeys [COTES et al., 1966]. This mechanism might really play a role in all the experiments refered above, but a definitive answer cannot be given unless the cells responsible for these phenomena are identified. In this connection, it is very interesting that in irradiated recipients the peritoneal macrophages of normal mice incubated with Shigella antigens were shown to be able to elicit antibody formation which could not be induced by antigen alone [GALLILY and FELDMAN, 1966]. The macrophages and not the contaminating lymphoid elements were found to be the effective cells. Undoubtedly, further studies of the relationship between macrophages and lymphoid cells will elucidate the relations between cells in both the induction of tolerance and immune reaction.

III. THE ROLE OF TOLERANCE

1. Genetic Determination of Immune Reaction

It has often been attributed to immunological tolerance that it is the mechanism protecting the organism from reacting immunologically to its own antigens ('self'). This is conceivable because tolerance has been anticipated as a hypothetical phenomenon to explain the non-reactivity to 'self' [BURNET and FENNER, 1949]. There is no other theory that would offer a plausible explanation of this phenomenon. The lack of an alternative cannot be ascribed only to the fact that the explanation of this non-reactivity by means of tolerance has been presented simultaneously with the questioning of its cause; it means that this explanation is satisfactory at the present state of knowledge. Views on how immunological tolerance works here keep on changing as new knowledge of the immunological mechanisms and the developments in other biological disciplines accumulate. A leading role in the formulation of the immunological concepts based on these developments was played in the past two decades by McFarland BURNET [BURNET and FENNER, 1949; BURNET, 1956, 1959, 1962, 1964], who made immunological tolerance and its role in non-reactivity to the organism's own antigens an integral part of these concepts.

The finding that even a typical adaptive process such as synthesis of the adaptive enzymes is determined at the level of the genetic code must have influenced speculations on the genetic determination of antibody formation. Furthermore, the observation of the differences in the primary structure of the antibody molecules which seems to be in direct association with their specificity has posed this question as a very pressing one. In the light of present knowledge of the relationship between the genetic code and protein-synthesis, it does not seem very likely that the different primary structure of antibodies might be caused by differences other than those in the genetic code. The theories attempting to explain the origin of antibody specificity by the direct or indirect effects of antigen on their synthesis taking place outside the genetic code, have little relevance in this situation. This does not mean that they have been proved to be incorrect. Ehrlich's theory of antibody formation anticipating the genetic determination of antibody formation did not seem to be relevant for a long time either. A convincing argument against this theory seemed to be Landsteiner's findings of immune reactions to different chemical haptens not encountered by the organism under normal conditions. The change in the general views presently held and the abandonment of the assumption of a direct genetic determination of antibody specificity can probably be brought about only by some new important discovery.

The first comprehensive theory based on these new facts and integrating all immunological problems was the clonal theory of antibody formation [Burnet, 1959; Lederberg, 1959]. Its principal value was to become the stimulus for a new approach to these problems. Its authors assume that there is only one locus for all antibodies. The great variability of this locus determining the occurrence of various antibodies is explained by its hypermutability in cells of the lymphoid tissues. Individual cell clones capable of immune reactions to different antigens would then primarily differ from each other by each having a different mutant of this gene. This concept is certainly not the strong point of this theory. Burnet [1964] made a modification in this theory by assuming that the cell clone is, to some limited extent, pluripotent.

An alternative to this concept is the view that each antibody is determined by an independent gene and that each somatic cell possesses genes for all antibodies. This has the advantage that such a constant ability of the organism as the immunological reaction to a wide range of antigens is not postulated to be determined by the random process of somatic cell mutation.

A considerable body of evidence is available that the genetic constitution of individuals of the same species affects their capacity for antibody formation. These data, however, apply mostly to the quantitative aspect of the process, i.e., the amount of antibodies formed by these animals against a given antigen. Nevertheless, it has been shown in the system of immune reactions to synthetic polypeptides that the quantitative differences among inbred mouse strains are apparently due to the differences in a single gene [McDewitt and Sela, 1965].

An exceptional observation was reported by Sobey and Sang [1954]. They found a male rabbit not producing antibodies against BSA even after intensive immunization; 10% of its offspring were non-reactive to BSA and the mode of inheritance seemed to show that this property was due to more than one gene. This finding would agree closely with the concept that each of these genes determined antibody formation against one determinant of BSA. The rabbit under study would lack the genetic information for antibody formation against all determinants of this antigen. The situation may, however, be much more complex, and an example (which I will give later on) will show that in this case a structural gene for antibody formation need not be involved. No progeny was obtained by mating non-reactive offspring of this rabbit. SOBEY et al. [1966] observed a similar non-reactivity in a male mouse which also proved to be determined polygenically. In this case, they succeeded in establishing a line from the progeny of this male; the line is being selected for this character, but is not yet homogeneous.

PINCHUK and MAURER [1965] found that members of three out of seven inbred strains of mice reacted by antibody formation against synthetic polypeptide-terpolymer $glu_{59}lys_{38}ala_5$. Either all the animals of a given strain reacted or else none of them did. In a random bred albino 'Swiss mice' strain some animals were capable of reaction while others were not. It has been shown by mating that the capacity for antibody formation is inherited as a dominant Mendelian factor. A similar genetic dependence for the inheritance of the capacity for immune reactions to synthetic polypeptides has been found in two inbred strains of guinea-pigs [BEN-EFRAIM and MAURER, 1966; BEN-EFRAIM et al., 1967].

The possible participation of more than one gene and not of the alleles of one locus in the configuration of the antibody combining sites has been shown by the results of ARQUILLA and FINN [1965]. They studied the configuration of the combining sites of antibodies against insulin in two inbred strains of guinea-pigs. These configurations differed in both strains: in most of the F_1 hybrids they did not differ significantly from the configurations of the parental strains, but in the F_2 generation different configurations appeared. No unequivocal conclusions can be drawn as yet from these findings because the divergent configurations might have been due to residual heterozygosity of the starting strains.

Very valuable insight into the mechanism of the genetic determination of immune reactions was provided by BENACERAFF and his associates. They observed that 30–40% of the guinea-pigs of the random bred Hartley strain were capable of reacting in an immune fashion to conjugates of poly-L-lysine with simple chemical haptens [KANTOR *et al.,* 1963; LEVINE *et al.,* 1963a]. Guinea-pigs of one inbred strain were capable of this reaction while those of another strain were not [LEVINE *et al.,* 1963b]. The capacity for the reaction proved to be determined by one dominant gene [LEVINE and BENACERAFF, 1964a]. These investigators at first assumed that immune-responder guinea-pigs had the capacity to metabolize poly-L-lysine in an appropriate manner. However, it appeared that the capacity of non-responder animals for enzymatic degradation of the poly-L-lysine was not impaired [LEVINE and BENACERAFF, 1964b]. A further analysis of this experimental model [GREEN *et al.,* 1966] revealed that the gene determining the reactivity to hapten-poly-L-lysine decides whether this substance is accepted by the animal as a complete antigen, or as a hapten only. The genetic determination of immune reaction will apparently be a complicated system. A significant role seems to be played by the not as yet more closely defined capacity to accept the introduced molecule as antigen. Studies have shown that even this capacity is determined genetically.

The evidence available confirms the genetic determination of antibody formation, but in no case has it been possible to prove that this determination is due to the presence or absence of the structural gene for the corresponding antibody. As this possibility has not been refuted, I will set forth the speculations based on this hypothesis.

In comparison with the clonal theory, the main drawback to the hypothesis that each somatic cell has the genes for all antibodies, which can be produced by the given organism, becomes obvious in explaining the induction of tolerance to autologous or foreign antigens. In BURNET and LEDERBERG's original clonal theory the induction of tolerance meant the elimination of the clone capable of immune reaction to the respective antigen. The other clones were not involved; antigens other than those towards which they were capable of reacting were indifferent to them. There was no difference whether the respective clone was destroyed during induction of tolerance, as anticipated in the original formulation of the theory, or whether it survived but its ability for immune reaction was inhibited [GORMAN and CHANDLER, 1964]. If each lymphoid cell has a genetic potential for immune reaction to any antigen, then the induction of tolerance to any antigen would potentially involve all lymphoid cells. The inhibitory process should then proceed in all cells potentially capable of the reaction. A similar idea is, at least implicitly, adopted in all instructive theories of antibody formation, but it cannot be denied that the explanation offered by the clonal theory is the most attractive, owing to its economy and simplicity.

On the basis of the hypothesis mentioned above one may raise the question whether non-reactivity to 'self' components is not caused by the primary lack of the structural or other genes regulating the formation of antibodies capable of reacting with indigenous components. It could be expected that the individuals whose fitness is threatened by an autoimmune reaction would be eliminated by natural selection, provided that the causative gene arises by mutation sufficiently rarely. This mechanism might be operative only if the antigen which would cause this autoimmune reaction were present in all or almost all individuals of the given species. Non-reactivity to individual specific antigens cannot, however, be explained in this way. These antigens differ in individual animals so that in each of them the immune reaction to other antigens must be eliminated. Moreover, the individual antigenic mosaicism is given by random combination of the genetic information from both parents. Insofar as immunological reactivity might be determined by independent genes for individual antibodies, even here the genetic information from each parent would be passed on by chance, and it would be difficult to imagine which mechanism might ensure that the gene for the particular individual antigen from one parent will not be transmitted simultaneously with the gene for the antibody against it from the other parent.

In the case of the clonal theory, assuming that the formation of different antibodies is determined by the same locus, the random course of the mutation process excludes the possibility that non-reactivity to the organism's own antigens might be due to lack of genetic information determining the formation of antibodies directed against these antigens.

It appears that non-reactivity to autologous antigens is brought about in a different way from that which occurs at the level of the basic genetic information. Whatever mechanism is responsible for this non-reactivity, it plays a significant role in the determination of the specificity of immunological reactivity of the organism, and this role is determined by the antigenic constitution of the organism. The antigenic make-up of the organism which is strictly genetically determined displays this influence on immunological reactivity. This aspect has been pointed out by CINADER [1960]. Non-reactivity to the organism's own antigenic determinants necessarily leads to a decrease or loss in antigenicity of foreign substances possessing the same determinants. The view that this mechanism plays a role in the determination of the specificity of immune reactivity was lent support by the findings on reactivity of mice to serum antigen MuB1 [CINADER and DUBISKI, 1964; CINADER et al., 1964, 1965]. Some inbred strains of mice possess this antigen and some lack it. When mice lacking this antigen are immunized with it, they form antibodies reacting not only with serum of mice possessing the antigen, but also with sera from many other species of rodents and other mammals. For example, all tested sera from some species, e. g., man, reacted with this antiserum, while sera from all individuals of other species did not. The same situation as in mice was observed in sheep and guinea-pigs: sera of some individuals reacted with this antiserum and some did not.

The authors explain these findings by assuming that in mice lacking MuB1 antigen the molecule carrying the respective antigenic specificity is, in fact, entirely absent. Such animals are not non-reactive to any part of this molecule, and when immunized with it, are capable of reacting with all its determinants. Therefore antibodies formed by them cross-react with a large number of antigens of other animal species.

We have seen that a foreign substance may be non-antigenic for two reasons. In addition to the possibility mentioned, namely that the potential for immune reactivity determined by inheritance is reduced by tolerance to autologous substances, there is a possibility that such a potential against the given substance is not present at all. These two cases could easily be distinguished by mating homozygous individuals, one capable of reaction and the other not. If non-reactivity to a certain substance is determined by its being a self component of the organism, then the heterozygous offspring from this mating will not be capable of immune reaction (Fig. 10). Its non-reactivity is due to the fact that it inherited the gene for this substance from one of its parents. Since the antigenic features are co-dominant, they produce a product of this gene and the respective substance becomes the indigenous substance of the body and hence non-antigenic. An example of such a situation are individual antigens responsible for tissue incompatibility. Members of the first filial generation produced by mating individuals from two different inbred strains are not capable of immune reaction to antigens of either parent. They are heterozygous in the genes for the antigens in which both strains differ. Hence they possess all antigens present in both strains and all these antigens are therefore 'self'. On the other hand, in all cases where this ability for antibody formation of certain

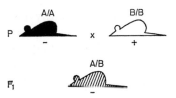

Fig. 10. Inheritance of reactivity to individual specific antigen caused by its presence or absence in the organism. A, B = allelic genes for individual specific antigens; + = ability to form anti-A antibodies; – = inability to form anti-A antibodies.

specificity appeared to be under direct genetic control, it was inherited as a dominant character. The particular individual is therefore capable of antibody synthesis, irrespective of being homo- or heterozygote for the respective gene. By mating individuals homozygous in their capacity for the formation of a certain antibody to individuals lacking this ability, an F₁ generation arises which is heterozygous for the given gene and hence capable of forming the antibody (Fig. 11).

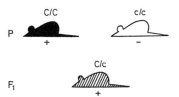

Fig. 11. Inheritance of genetically determined ability to form antibody of certain specificity. C = dominant gene determining the ability to form particular antibody; c = recessive gene determining the inability to form particular antibody; + = ability to form particular antibody; – = inability to form particular antibody.

2. Experimental Attempts to Demonstrate the Role of Immunological Tolerance as a Mechanism Involved in Non-Reactivity to the Organism's Own Components

The most convincing evidence for the view that non-reactivity to 'self' components develops as an adaptive process during early life as a result of the action of these components was provided by TRIPLETT [1962]. The hypophyses of embryos of the tree-frog *(Hyla regilla)* were extirpated and implanted temporarily in the dermis of other animals about two weeks old. When the donors reached metamorphic stage the explanted hypophyses were returned to them as dermal grafts. Since the hypophysis secretes a hormone which causes the dermal melanophores to expand, the hypophysectomized animals were light in colour. Within a few minutes after the grafting was accomplished, they turned dark and remained so if the graft was accepted. If the graft was rejected, they again became apparent albinos. The fate of the graft and the complete removal of the hypophysis were checked histologically 60 days after transplantation. In most cases, the hypophyseal grafts were rejected when they were returned to their original donors. To exclude the possibility that their specificity did not change as a result of culture in a temporary host, which might cause the rejection, Triplett (in another series of experiments) removed only part of the hypophysis, cultivated the extirpated hypophysis in a foreign host and thereafter transferred it back to the original donor. In this group, in no case were the grafts rejected. Autografts of the tail were also accepted in completely hypophysectomized animals, whereas the homografts were mostly rejected. This experiment furnishes evidence that hypophysectomy did not change the reactivity so as to bring about the rejection of grafts of any tissue.

Similarly, Vojtíšková and Poláčková [1966] attempted to demonstrate the ability for immune reaction to an organism's own antigen which usually does not elicit it. They used the sex-antigen (H-Y) in mice. They tried to block its development by castration of males of the C57Bl/6 strain within 48 h of birth, but this treatment led only to a decrease, not a complete suppression, of H-Y antigen in the castrated males. Their grafts survived on females of the same strain significantly longer (average 50.0 ± 6.3 days) than those from control males (27.2 ± 1.1 days) of the same age (10–11 weeks), but were finally rejected in most cases. The behaviour of these grafts resembled the survival of grafts from young, antigenically immature males. Grafts from 10-day-old males survived for 51.7 ± 2.9 days and from 2-day-old males 75.9 ± 4.6 days. The permanent survival of skin grafts from the normal males suggested that the castrated males were non-reactive towards H-Y antigen.

Further experiments carried out to demonstrate the role of tolerance in non-reactivity to autologous antigens started from a different point, i. e., the autoimmune lesions of the organs produced by immunization with extract from the respective organ incorporated in complete

Freund's adjuvant. In addition to the pathologic lesions, autoimmune reactions of both delayed-type hypersensitivity and circulating antibodies are demonstrable in such syndromes. The pathogenetic relationship of this immune reaction to the organ lesions has been confirmed in experimental allergic encephalomyelitis by the adoptive transfer of lymphoid cells from immunized animals [PATERSON, 1960; STONE, 1961]. The reactivity to these antigens is explained by the hypothesis according to which the antigens involved, under normal conditions, do not come in contact with cells responsible for an immune reaction. The outcome of their isolation is that in the early developmental stages they do not elicit non-reactivity to themselves as do other autoantigens which reach these cells. The isolation of these presumably non-tolerated antigens is the reason why they do not elicit an autoimmune reaction in adult life in spite of being antigenic. In this case, an afferent inhibition of the immune reaction may be involved.

PATERSON [1958] tried to change this situation by injecting newborn rats with nervous tissue. He anticipated that these organ antigens might thus come in contact with the lymphoid tissue and might be capable of eliciting autotolerance. Animals treated in this way did not in fact display signs of allergic encephalomyelitis after immunization with nervous tissue in complete Freund's adjuvant.

In our Institute a similar model was used: experimental allergic aspermatogenesis which can be induced by immunization with testicular antigen in complete Freund's adjuvant. Postnatal injections of antigen were capable of suppressing or reducing the development of allergic aspermatogenesis in guinea-pigs after challenge with antigen in complete Freund's adjuvant when they reached immunological maturity [CHUTNÁ et al., 1962; VOJTÍŠKOVÁ et al., 1962]. The advantage of this model seemed to be that the antigen responsible for the induction of the autoimmune syndrome was absent in sexually immature animals [KATSH, 1960; BISHOP et al., 1961]. However, it appeared to be present there, though in lower concentrations than in mature animals [POKORNÁ and VOJTÍŠKOVÁ, 1964b].

Some doubt has been cast on the interpretation of these results as immunological tolerance to the organism's own antigens by the findings that following challenge with antigen from nervous tissue in Freund's adjuvant complement-fixing antibodies can be demonstrated in neonatally injected rats, whose capacity for the development of allergic encephalomyelitis has been decreased [PATERSON and HARWIN, 1962]. Since serum of immune rats containing these antibodies was capable of preventing or suppressing allergic encephalomyelitis after passive transfer to sensitized animals [PATERSON *et al.*, 1961; PATERSON and HARWIN, 1963], the mechanism of suppression of allergic encephalomyelitis following neonatal injection of antigen became uncertain.

A similar situation has been observed with allergic aspermatogenesis. Its occurrence has been prevented by the administration of testicular antigen in saline before challenge with antigen incorporated in complete Freund's adjuvant [CHUTNÁ and RYCHLÍKOVÁ, 1964a]. The possibility of transferring this effect passively with serum has not been clearly demonstrated. The immune sera did suppress the development of allergic aspermatogenesis, but a similar effect was also displayed by sera from normal animals [POKORNÁ and VOJTÍŠKOVÁ, 1964c, 1966]. However, the antisera prepared by immunization with testicular antigen without adjuvant were capable of protecting testicular cells *in vitro* from the damaging effects of circulating cytotoxic antibodies appearing after immunization with antigen in complete Freund's adjuvant [CHUTNÁ and RYCHLÍKOVÁ, 1964b].

The possibility is not excluded that the suppression observed after postnatal injection of antigen is, at least in part, due to tolerance. This is suggested by the results of CHUTNÁ and RYCHLÍKOVÁ [1966] showing that large doses of testicular antigen administered after immunization in complete Freund's adjuvant suppress the immune reaction and the development of the damage to the testes. The suppression achieved in this way involves all components of the immune reaction and does not seem to be the outcome of desensitization only. However, the uncertainties in explaining the mechanism involved in these phenomena make it impossible to use the above results as supporting evidence for the question discussed here.

3. Occurrence of Autoimmune Reactions

The examples given here of experimental autoimmune syndromes are thus explained not as a failure of the mechanism involved in non-reactivity to 'self' components but as the result of the isolation of these substances which therefore cannot induce non-reactivity. In human pathology, the existence of autoimmune antibodies is described which cannot be explained in this way, because the cells carrying the respective antigens are in intimate contact with the lymphoid tissue; I am thinking of the occurrence of autoantibodies against erythrocytes which are an ideal cellular object for serological analyses. It is not important whether or not these antibodies are the primary cause of the pathological states in which they are mainly detected. It is essential that this is a well-documented occurrence of autoantibodies directed against the antigen of cells appearing in the organism at such sites where foreign antigens or cells carrying them elicit an immune reaction. If the immune reaction towards such own antigens takes place, the mechanism must have failed which is, under normal conditions, involved in non-reactivity to them. However, in most humans autohaemagglutinins are present which are capable of agglutinating their own erythrocytes, not at body temperature, but at low temperatures. This property is certainly not insignificant, but the fact that these autoantibodies occur regularly is of special relevance to the subject in hand.

MILGROM et al. [1957] made an important contribution to the understanding of autoantibodies occurring regularly in normal individuals. They have reported that the fluid from mechanically produced skin blisters in humans contained group isoagglutinins and autohaemagglutinins reacting not only at 4 °C and room temperature, but also at 37 °C, though this latter reaction was weaker. Auto-haemagglutinins were demonstrated in all individuals tested. They were most easily detectable in fresh blister fluid. In older blisters their titre decreased and eventually they disappeared, and only natural group isoagglutinins remained in the fluid. This finding has been confirmed by BURGIO and SEVERI [1963, 1964, 1965], who used can-tharidin adhesive plaster to produce skin blisters. Since in this case it took a longer time before a blister developed, the fluid was collected after 18–20 h. This might have been the reason why autoagglutinins could not be detected in all individuals examined (they were found in 77% of the cases.) The antibody nature of these autohaemagglutinins was proved by GENOVA and VACCARO [1964] by the immunofluo-rescence technique. Further knowledge of them is, unfortunately, limited. For example, it is not known what their biological activity is, how they appear in the blister fluid or why they are absent in serum. Nevertheless, this finding supports the view that autoantibody formation is not an exceptional phenomenon confined to pathological states, but that it may occur generally in normal individuals.

There are some autoimmune reactions that probably occur relatively frequently. Autoimmune reactions similar to those evoked by immunization with homo- or autologous organ substances incorporated in complete Freund's adjuvant may also be produced by material from the corresponding organs of members of a foreign species [KAPLAN, 1958; KAPLAN and CRAIG, 1963; WITEBSKY and ROSE, 1959; JOHNSTON et al., 1963; KIES, 1965] and even without adjuvant [TERPLAN et al., 1960]. Such heterologous antigens may lead both to the formation of autoantibodies and the lesions in the respective organ of immunized animals. Heterologous antigens not only cross-react with autologous substances, but are capable of inducing autoimmune reactions better than autoantigens. Immunization with organ antigens from animals of a foreign species is possible only under experimental conditions. From the point of view of induction of an autoimmune reaction, cross-reactivity between antigens of an immunized organism and microbial antigens is more important. That such a sharing of antigens may result in the occurrence of an autoimmune reaction has been shown in a number of cases. In the first place, it is the formation of autoantibodies against heart antigens in rabbits induced by streptococcal antigen [KAPLAN, 1963; KAPLAN and SUCHY, 1964; KAPLAN and SVEC, 1964]. Another example is cross-reactivity of E.coli with cells of gastric mucosa which may also give rise to autoantibodies and possibly to organ lesions [HOLBOROW et al., 1963; PERLMANN et al., 1965]. That in this case antigens of intestinal bacteria deposited in the tissue are not involved is proved by the localization of the organ antigen and the possibility of demonstrating it in cells of the gastro-intestinal tract of germ-free animals. Finally, a well demonstrated example of autoantibody formation elicited by microbial antigens are autoantibodies against rabbit liver and kidneys induced by infection with Eimeria stiediae [ASHERSON and ROSE, 1963].

After discussing the significance of cold agglutinins in understanding the limits and the mechanism of autoimmune reactions I would like to point out that they increase in titre as a result of viral pneumonia. In this connection, I would like to recall the finding of cold autohaemagglutinins in rabbits following immunization with homologous erythrocytes (OVARY and SPIEGELMAN. 1965],

All these findings are reminiscent of the abolition of tolerance to heterologous serum proteins by means of cross-reacting serum proteins of another species or tolerated antigen conjugated to simple haptens [CINADER and DUBERT, 1955, 1956; WEIGLE, 1961, 1962]. The similarity is accentuated by the observation that the formation of autoimmune antibodies and the lesions to the testes could be elicited without adjuvant with homologous organ antigens conjugated to sulphanilic acid [POKORNÁ and VOJTÍŠKOVÁ, 1964a].

Similar results were obtained by WEIGLE [1965 b]. In rabbits, the injection of soluble homologous thyroglobulin conjugated simultaneously to arsanilic and sulphanilic acid resulted in the formation of circulating antibodies against native thyroglobulin and lesions to the thyroid. These animals reacted by an increased level of antibodies when injected with native thyroglobulin, which does not induce an immune reaction in normal rabbits. On repeating the injections of native thyroglobulin, the antibody response decreased, and some rabbits formed no antibodies following a third injection of native thyroglobulin. It is interesting that the lesions to the thyroids were present in the largest percentage of rabbits in the group examined after the third injection of native thyroglobulin.

An objection might be raised that in the above cases autoantigens are involved to which no tolerance has been induced. Evidence is, however, available that antibodies against autologous erythrocytes may arise by this mechanism for which this explanation does not hold. It has been shown by BUSSARD and HUYNH [1960] that during short-term cultivation the lymph node cells from rabbits intensively immunized with sheep erythrocytes produced antibodies capable of binding onto autologous erythrocytes. This has been confirmed by INGRAHAM and BUSSARD [1964]. Using the method of localized haemolysis in gel they found that cells lysing their own erythrocytes were present in the regional lymph nodes of rabbits immunized with sheep erythrocytes.

Evidence of autoantibody formation following immunization with heterologous antigens has also been provided with some chemically defined components. After immunization of rabbits with porcine lactoso-dehydrogenase in complete Freund's adjuvant RAJEWSKY [1966] demonstrated antibodies reacting with the corresponding, even autologous, rabbit enzyme.

During immunization of rabbits with various heterologous cytochromes c, performed without adjuvant but either with a solution of the enzyme or its conjugate to acetyl-BGG, NISONOFF et al. [1967] obtained antibodies reacting with rabbit enzyme, even autologous one.

The above results are very important because the enzymes involved occur in almost all tissues of the organism, quite certainly in cells forming antibodies against them, and possibly also in other cells participating in the immune reaction.

In the case of autoantibodies elicited by cross-reactions with bacterial antigen it should be emphasized that the possibility is to be excluded that the autoimmune reaction is directed against microbial antigens localized in the tissues. In experiments with well-defined 'self' components it should be borne in mind that the organism's own substance may be denatured during preparation. The altered 'self' components may become antigenic for the organism. MILGROM and WITEBSKY [1960] showed that rabbits immunized with autologous γ-globulin isolated by fractionation with ammonium-sulphate produced antibodies reacting with the autologous preparation used for immunization in a considerably lower titre than with human γ-globulin. The authors assumed that the antigenicity of the own γ-globulin was due to moderate denaturation during preparation. These results were confirmed for both rabbits and guinea-pigs by McCLUS-KEY et al. [1962] who further analysed the conditions of denaturation endowing autologous γ-globulins with autoantigenicity. However, they did not find any reaction with autologous native γ-globulin in such immune animals nor could they induce an autoimmune reaction by it. This mechanism is probably responsible for the occurrence of so-called anti-antibodies. They are antibodies reacting with the autologous γ-globulin modified by the binding to antigen, but not with free γ-globulin. Their presence has been demonstrated: (a) in man [MILGROM et al., 1956a]; (b) in rabbits [MILGROM, 1962].

In addition to the findings of BUSSARD and his associates on autoimmunity to autologous erythrocytes induced by heterologous erythrocytes, the possible role of this mechanism is most convincingly excluded by the results of RAJEWSKY. He showed that antibodies against lactoso-dehydrogenase formed in rabbits were bound to this enzyme in the blood. In both these cases, it seems very unlikely that autologous substances reacting with antibodies would be denatured.

4. Possible Mechanisms Involved in Non-Reactivity to Own Components

In the paragraph on the genetic determination of antibody formation, evidence has been presented suggesting that non-reactivity to indigenous substances is, at least as regards the individual specific antigens, an acquired phenomenon not determined genetically. I have left the way open for the possibility of a genetic determination of the non-reactivity to the species specific antigens. Natural selection might, in fact, here, lead to the elimination of individuals that would be at a disadvantage as a result of autoimmune reactions. If non-reactivity to various 'self' components were effected through this dual mechanism, it might be expected that its failure would take place more readily in the case of individual specific antigens where the immune reaction is genetically determined, but its realization is prevented. The frequent observations of individual specificity of autoantibodies in haemolytic anaemia [DACIE, 1965] would be in agreement with this view. Individual antigens of erythrocytes are the best known system of this category of antigens and hence this finding is of considerable importance. Organ antigens may also display individual specificity [ROSE et al., 1960] and the individual specificity of the γ-globulin molecule is well known [OUDIN, 1966]. Thus it is possible that the lesions produced in experimental autoallergic syndromes and antibodies detectable in other autoimmune reactions might be directed against autologous individual specific organ antigens. Evidence for this view is lacking so far, but neither have contrary results been obtained. If there is a mechanism other than the genetic one which elicits non-reactivity to certain 'self' substances, i.e., the individual specific ones, it seems unlikely that it would not evoke non-reactivity to all the organism's own substances. It follows that natural selection operating on the basis of the damage to the individual by an autoimmune reaction could not take effect here.

In the preceding paragraph evidence has been presented that the autoimmune reaction is not an exceptional event. It cannot be expected, and has not been observed, that such reactions might frequently result in lesions to the organism. The existence of a pathological condition where an autoimmune reaction might probably primarily or secondarily cause damage is rare. The situation encountered here seems to suggest that the organism eliminates those autoimmune reactions that are dangerous to it and is not concerned with those not threatening it. It is, of course, difficult to imagine how discrimination would be ensured on the basis of this criterion. If any mechanism operates to achieve this aim, it must be based on a different principle. Moreover, it cannot be expected that the same types of reaction would be of equal danger to various tissues and cells.

Now I would like to turn my attention to the mechanism which might play a role in bringing about the form of reduced immune reactivity to indigenous components which is observed in higher animals. Since absolute non-reactivity is not obviously involved, the possibility must be considered whether autoimmune reactions occurring under normal conditions might not themselves have been the mechanism producing the limited immune reaction to 'self' components. Evidence has been provided that in experimental autoallergic syndromes some types of antibody may interfere with other types of immune reaction which cause the tissue lesions and thus may act protectively. It is of interest that these types of antibody occur in allergic encephalomyelitis and aspermatogenesis following immunization of animals with tissue antigens alone whereas the use of complete Freund's adjuvant, leads to damage to the target tissue.

With organ-isolated antigens, the circulating antibodies might be the mechanism preventing the development of a dangerous autoimmune reaction evoked by escape of antigen from this isolation.

These as well as other possibilities are only hypothetical. No evidence is available that some immunosuppressive mechanisms might really operate as a factor reducing the development of autoimmunity.

Delayed hypersensitivity seems to be the most important component eliciting autoallergic lesions in experimental syndromes and possibly in diseases in which autoimmunity is the pathogenetic factor [Roitt and Doniach, 1967]. In immune deviation its reduction or suppression takes place while some other types of antibody are formed which might possibly function as protective antibodies. The consideration seems to be justified that immune deviation might play a role as a mechanism preventing the development of autoimmune reactions [Asherson, 1967], especially those that are dangerous to the organism. The question is whether immune deviation is not involved when another defence line, be it the organ isolation of antigen, autotolerance or some other factor, broke down. It is also possible that some forms of autoimmune reactions are the manifestation of incomplete autotolerance.

Experiments trying to demonstrate that non-reactivity to the body's own components is determined by tolerance to them, by means of induction of tolerance to organ antigens responsible for experimental allergic encephalomyelitis and aspermatogenesis, are not convincing enough. They provide only indirect evidence, and the kind of mechanism involved in the suppression obtained in this way is not known so far. Moreover, the assumption that these substances do not induce tolerance towards themselves, because they are separated from cells responsible for antibody formation, is uncertain. In this connection I would like to draw attention to another aspect of this phenomenon. It is difficult to exclude the possibility that the 'self' components used for such immunizations are damaged during preparation and that these denatured components are actually responsible for the induction of an autoimmune syndrome. With regard to the possibility of inducing the formation of autoantibodies even after immunization with these preparations without complete Freund's adjuvant it appears that the production of the pathological lesions when an adjuvant has been used for immunization, might be due to an increase in the intensity of immune reactions rather than to a change in their nature. The adjuvant itself does not seem to be indispensable in the sense that it would only in itself make an antigen from the preparation incapable of eliciting an immune reaction as is the case, for example, with BGG devoid of adjuvanticity for mice by ultracentrifugation [DRESSER, 1961a]. This view on the quantitative rather than qualitative influence of an adjuvant on the developement of autoallergic syndromes is supported by the finding that the preparation from guinea-pig testes administered without complete adjuvant produces damage to spermatogenesis in some animals, though of a low degree [POKORNÁ and VOJTÍŠKOVÁ, 1964a].

Although the finding on non-reactivity to indigenous hypophysis, which has been removed from the organism in the embryonic stage, [TRIPLETT, 1962] is convincing evidence for the role of antigen in the induction of non-reactivity to the organism's own components, it does not answer the question as to which mechanism is responsible for it. The age at which this takes place seems to suggest that the mechanism involved might be immunological tolerance.

The view that immunological tolerance is the mechanism responsible for this seems to be supported by a striking similarity between the possibility of abolishing immunological tolerance and eliciting the development of autoimmune reactions by cross-reactive antigens. In both cases, such reactions are not very strong. With the tolerance states, it is obviously possible to overcome the suppression and induce antibody formation, but a major part of tolerance persists. If the same mechanism plays a role in the induction of an autoimmune reaction, this might explain why these reactions are relatively weak. Moreover, the presence of tolerated antigen may prevent escape from tolerance, or possibly re-induce it [WEIGLE, 1964b].

It follows from these facts that the idea that non-reactivity to 'self' components is produced by autotolerance explains the given situation best, but it must be kept in mind that this is a hypothesis only which requires experimental verification.

IV. CONCLUDING REMARKS

Many questions concerning the mechanism and the biological role of immunological tolerance remain unanswered. One of those which cannot be regarded as being satisfactorily answered is the existence of tolerance as a phenomenon caused by a certain mechanism. The discovery of other types of the suppression states of immune reactions caused by a different mechanism contributed very much to our knowledge of these problems. The relationships between these different phenomena still await further elucidation. All these suppression states of immune reaction and especially immunological tolerance have become an integral and important part of general immunology. In addition to the theoretical significance, the question of specific suppression of the immune reactions has important practical aspects. Tissue incompatibility due to transplantation immunity is at the present time the main obstacle to therapeutic tissue transplantations. This involves the possibility of substituting an organ damaged by injury or a pathological process or to introduce functionally competent cells into an organism incapable of synthesizing a certain enzyme, hormone or another effective substance as a result of an inherited or acquired defect. This obstacle is felt to be the more serious as the technical difficulties which might impede transplantation in surgery have been virtually overcome.

However, the practical problems associated with the suppression of immune reactions are not exhausted by this. Even in the domain where immunity seems to be a very useful defence mechanism of the organism, i.e. immunity to infection, there are many reactions (especially of the hypersensitivity type) where an inhibition would be desirable. It is, however, doubtful whether in this domain immunological tolerance is desirable. Other treatments leading to specific inhibition of certain types of immune reactions only may be more helpful and probably more easily induced here. It is now necessary to mention the problem of allergy. I do not feel competent to deal with the immunological questions of therapy or prevention of allergic conditions. I wish only to emphasize that this field is of equal importance as the whole question of transplantation in the application of new facts on the inhibition states of immune reaction. Its long immunological tradition represents a significant source of valuable knowledge and stimuli also for basic immunological research.

Although my attention is centred upon immunological tolerance, or, maybe for just that reason, I realize how utterly reckless it would be to look for the suppression of undesirable immune reactions only in this field. A very useful practical contribution has recently been made by using antibodies for immunosuppression. I have in mind the prevention of haemolytic disease in newborns by means of anti-Rh serum administered passively to pregnant women at the time of expected sensitization with erythrocytes from the foetus [CLARKE, 1966]. From the point of view of practical application, it makes no difference whether the antibodies administered act by removing the foetal erythrocytes from the circulation and thus mediate the suppression of immune reaction at the afferent level, or whether they act in a different way.

The immunological relationships between mother and foetus are also a good example of the role played by both tolerance and other types of immunological non-reactivity in the spheres that at first sight seem to be distantly related. The questions of tolerance induced by maternal antigens in the foetus are very close to my subject. A relatively low incidence of erythroblastosis foetalis produced by Rh-incompatibility between mother and foetus raised the question of whether this might not be due to tolerance of the mother acquired during the intrauterine life toward Rh+ antigen of her mother. However, the frequency of haemolytic disease of newborns appeared not to correlate with Rh antigens of their grandmothers [BOOTH et al., 1953; OWEN et al., 1954; WARD et al., 1957]. Despite this, a certain degree of tolerance to maternal antigens may be induced because the daughters of Rh— mothers form anti-Rh antibodies during pregnancy more frequently than daughters of Rh+ mothers [OWEN et al., 1954]. The conditions for the induction of tolerance to antigens of maternal erythrocytes are present. Passage of erythrocytes from foetus to mother has been demonstrated, and thus a reverse passage is practically certain. It might therefore be expected that tolerance to antigens of the ABO system can also be induced. Natural anti-A and anti-B antibodies seemed to be a very suitable indicator of this state. WICHER and WOZNICZKO-ORLOWSKA [1960] and later MAYEDA [1966] found no difference in the titres of these natural haemagglutinins depending on the blood group of the mother. The individuals they tested were 18–22 years old; it might be claimed that tolerance has disappeared in them. We therefore examined 6-month-old children, as we supposed that if tolerance were induced in them it would be easiest to detect [HRABA et al., 1962]. Even in this case no difference was found in the onset of anti-A haemagglutinin formation or titre depending on whether or not the mother possessed this antigen. JAKOBOWICZ et al., [1959] did observe a difference in their experiments. They ana-lysed the titres of anti-A haemolysins in army trainees of the O-group after immunization with tetanus toxoid containing the A substance. The titre of this antibody was significantly higher in sons of O-group moth-ers than in sons of A-group mothers. This difference could be observed with natural haemolysins already before immunization with toxoid.

These results suggest that the placental barrier is not entirely imper-meable and that a certain degree of tolerance to maternal antigens can be induced in the foetus. As far as the induction of transplantation tolerance to maternal antigens is concerned, it seemed to be a rare phenomenon under normal conditions [BILLINGHAM et al., 1956a; BILLINGHAM, 1964]. However, this does not appear to be the case. When the fate of skin grafts transferred from rabbit father and mother to a newborn rabbit was followed, the survival of maternal grafts was significantly longer than that of paternal ones [IVÁNYI and DÉMANT, 1965; DÉMANT et al., 1966]. It is very likely that a longer survival of maternal grafts is due to tolerance to their antigens, although this conclusion requires further verification. The difference between these findings and the earlier observations in which this phenomenon has not been found may be explained by the fact that in earlier experiments the transplantation was performed at a later age. If chimaerism of maternal cells in the foetus has not been established, and this is very likely, the tolerance induced will be short-term; then there is more hope of detecting it shortly after birth. Moreover, even though tests are made immediately after birth, the prolongation in the graft sur-vival is not comparable to the situation encountered in strong states of tolerance. The amount of antigen passing through the placenta under normal conditions may not be sufficient to induce strong tol-erance. Damage to this barrier by irradiation results in strong tolerance in the majority of offspring [LENGEROVÁ, 1957].

In the immunological relationship between foetus and mother a situation exists which is difficult to reconcile with the ideas on toler-ance. The molecules of γ-globulin carrying Gm antigen can pass

through the placenta in both directions in man. It might be expected
that tolerance to this maternal antigen will be induced in children.
This expectation has not been fulfilled; on the contrary, the children
were found to possess a high incidence of antibodies against the
maternal Gm factor which appear spontaneously during the first year
of life [SPEISER, 1963; SPEISER and MICKERTS, 1964; STEINBERG and
WILSON, 1963; WILSON and STEINBERG, 1965; SANDER and STICHNOT,
1963; FUDENBERG and FUDENBERG, 1964]. This phenomenon, considered from the point of view of tolerance, resembles spontaneous
onset of the immune reaction as observed in mice after the disappearance of tolerance to heterologous serum proteins and pneumococcal polysaccharides. The other possibility is that the form of antigen
could be at play here. Precipitates of HSA with rabbit anti-HSA antibodies were shown to induce immunity instead of tolerance in newborn
rabbits [CHUTNÁ and HRABA, 1962]. It may well be the case that maternal antibodies bind with some antigen in the foetus and thus become the stimulus for antibody formation. In this connection, I would
like to draw attention to frequent autospecificity of the rheumatoid
factor in the Gm system [KUNKEL and TAN, 1964]. It would be interesting to know whether these two phenomena were somehow associated. At any rate, it can be anticipated that this finding, owing to
its non-orthodoxy, may be the stimulus for the study of some unexpected aspects of tolerance.

The relationship between mother and foetus is also interesting from
an immunological point of view, and its understanding will certainly
also be important for practical purposes. The foetus is virtually a
physiological graft which, unlike other allogeneic grafts, does not induce a transplantation immune reaction. It is interesting that repeated
pregnancies result in a decrease of the reactivity to paternal antigens
in the mother. This has been discovered by means of tumor [BREYERE
and BARRETT, 1960 a, 1961] and skin grafts [PREHN, 1960; BREYERE
and BARRETT, 1960 b]. With mouse sex-antigen H-Y, it has been shown
that the cause of the suppression of the reaction towards this antigen
need not be only the pregnancy itself, but also the ejaculate [LEN-
GEROVÁ and VOJTÍŠKOVÁ, 1962, 1963]. Although with this antigen,
immunological tolerance is probably responsible for the graft survival
in this situation, other suppression mechanisms may be involved when
other antigens are used. The effect observed may not explain immunological non-reactivity of the mother towards the foetus as the suppression of immunological reactivity is generally too weak.

The placental barrier may prevent the passage of cells and of some substances, but the immune reaction of the mother may be elicited by direct contact of her elements with the foetal membranes of amniotic origin. Although it has been impossible to demonstrate the paternal antigens in the foetal part of the placenta when there was a weak antigenic difference between father and mother [HAŠKOVÁ, 1961, 1962, 1963], with a strong antigenic difference the paternal antigens were detected [SIMMONS and RUSSELL, 1962; UHR and ANDERSON, 1962; HAŠKOVÁ, 1963]. Therefore the absence of the paternal antigens in the foetal membranes cannot offer an explanation of the mother's non-reactivity to the foetus, except in the case where cells of the foetal membranes, which are in direct contact with the maternal tissues, do not possess the paternal antigens. This explanation is only speculative and an answer to this question is to be sought in further experiments.

The abolition of tolerance with a cross-reactive antigen appears to be a crucial point in understanding the mechanism of tolerance and perhaps the cause of autoimmune reactions. From a practical point of view, it may be important to prevent this escape in the states of tolerance which are desirable, e. g., transplantation tolerance and autotolerance. In clinical pratice cases are known where the abolition of tolerance would probably be very desirable. Tolerance can be induced readily to specific tumor antigens [KOLDOVSKÝ and SVOBODA, 1962; KOLDOVSKÝ, 1967] and this situation may probably be encountered in human tumor diseases. The reaction towards these antigens would, however, be most useful from a therapeutic point of view, and hence in this case the abolition of tolerance might be of definite practical importance.

A number of other possible practical applications of the suppression of immune reactions may be found. Unfortunately, only a few of them have been realized so far. Nevertheless, I hope that the situation will change in the near future.

REFERENCES

ADA, G. L.; NOSSAL, G. J. V. and AUSTIN, C. M.: Studies on the nature of immunogenicity employing soluble and particulate bacterial proteins; in Molecular and Cellular Basis of Antibody Formation, p. 31 (Publ. House Czech. Acad. Sci., Prague 1965a).

ADA, G. L.; NOSSAL, G. J. V. and PYE, J.: Antigens in immunity. XI. The uptake of antigen in animals previously rendered immunologically tolerant. Austr. J. exp. Biol. med. Sci. 43: 337–344 (1965b).

ADLER, F. L.: Competition of antigens. Progr. Allergy, vol. 8, pp. 41–57 (Karger, Basel/New York 1964).

ALBRIGHT, J. F. and EVANS, T. W.: Influence of antigen dosage on kinetics of hemagglutinating antibody production. J. Immunol. 95: 368–377 (1965).

ALBRIGHT, J. F. and MAKINODAN, T.: Dynamics of expression of competence of antibody-producing cells; in Molecular and Cellular Basis of Antibody Formation, p. 427 (Publ. House Czech. Acad. Sci., Prague 1965).

ANDERSON, D.; BILLINGHAM, R. E.; LAMPKIN, G. H. and MEDAWAR, P. B.: The use of skin grafting to distinguish between monozygotic and dizygotic twins in cattle. Heredity 5: 379–397 (1951).

ARGYRIS, B. F.: Acquired tolerance to skin grafts in mice. I. Histological analysis of lymphoid tissue before, during and after the loss of tolerance. J. exp. Med. 117: 543–560 (1963).

ARGYRIS, B. F.: Adoptive tolerance transferred by bone marrow, spleen, lymph node or thymus cells. J. Immunol. 96: 273–278 (1966).

ARIMA, J.; YAMAMOTO, K.; MORIKAWA, K. et TAKAHASHI, Y.: Sur le développement tardif de l'allergie tuberculeuse chez le cobaye à la suite de l'inoculation intraveineuse de BCG. C. R. Soc. Biol. 152: 1292–1295 (1958).

ARNASON, B. G.; JANKOVIĆ, B. D.; WAKSMAN, B. H. and WENNERSTEN, CH.: Role of the thymus in immune reactions in rats. II. Suppressive effect of thymectomy at birth on reactions of delayed (cellular) hypersensitivity and the circulating small lymphocyte. J. exp. Med. 116: 177–186 (1962).

ARQUILLA, E. R. and FINN, J.: Genetic control of combining sites of insulin antibodies produced by guinea pigs. J. exp. Med. 122: 771–784 (1965).

ASHERSON, G. L.: Selective and specific inhibition of 24 h skin reactions in the guinea-pig. II. The mechanism of immune deviation. Immunology, Lond. 10: 179–186 (1966).

ASHERSON, G. L.: Antigen-mediated depression of delayed hypersensitivity. Brit. med. Bull. 23: 24–29 (1967).

ASHERSON, G. L. and ROSE, M. E.: Autoantibody production in rabbits. III. The effect of infection with Eimeria stiedae and its relation to natural antibody. Immunology, Lond. 6: 207–216 (1963).

Asherson, G. L. and Stone, S. H.: Selective and specific inhibition of 24 h skin reactions in the guinea pigs. I. Immune deviation: description of the phenomenon and the effect of splenectomy. Immunology, Lond. 9: 205–217 (1965).

Austin, C. M. and Nossal, G. J. V.: Mechanism of induction of immunological tolerance. III. Cross-tolerance amongst flagellar antigens. Austr. J. exp. Biol. med. Sci. 44: 341–353 (1966).

Barnes, D. W. H.; Ilbery, P. L.T. and Loutit, J. F.: Avoidance of 'secondary disease' in radiation chimaeras. Nature, Lond. 181: 488 (1958).

Barrett, M. K. and Breyere, E. J.: Strain-specific tolerance to skin or tumor homografts in postpartum mice; in Mechanisms of Immunological Tolerance, p. 347 (Publ. House Czech. Acad. Sci., Prague 1962).

Battisto, J. R. and Bloom, B. R.: Dual immunological unresponsiveness induced by cell membrane coupled hapten or antigen. Nature, Lond. 212: 156–157 (1966).

Battisto, J.R. and Chase, M. W.: Immunological unresponsiveness to sensitization with simple chemical compounds. A search for antibody-absorbing depots of allergen. J. exp. Med. 118: 1021–1035 (1963).

Battisto, J. R. and Chase, M. W.: Induced unresponsiveness to simple allergenic chemicals. II. Independence of delayed-type hypersensitivity and formation of circulating antibody. J. exp. Med. 121: 591–606 (1965).

Battisto, J. R. and Miller, J.: Immunological unresponsiveness produced in adult guinea pigs by parenteral introduction of minute quantities of hapten or protein antigen. Proc. Soc. exp. Biol., N. Y. 111: 111–115 (1962).

Bekkum, D. W. van: Tolerance of donor cells towards the host in radiation chimeras; in Mechanisms of Immunological Tolerance, p. 385 (Publ. House Czech. Acad. Sci., Prague 1962).

Bekkum, D. W. van: Determination of specific immunological tolerance in radiation chimeras. Transplantation 1: 39–57 (1963).

Ben-Efraim, S.; Fuchs, S. and Sela, M.: Differences in immune response to synthetic antigens in two inbred-strains of guinea pigs. Immunology 12: (in press 1967).

Ben-Efraim, S. and Maurer, P.H.: Immune response to polypeptides (poly-α-amino acids) in inbred guinea-pigs. J. Immunol. 97: 577–586 (1966).

Benirschke, K.; Anderson, J. M. and Brownhill, L.E.: Marrow chimerism in marmosets. Science 138: 513–515 (1962).

Billingham, R. E.: Transplantation immunity and the maternal-fetal relationship. Trans. & Stud. College of Physicians, Philadelphia, ser. 4, 31: 187–203 (1964).

Billingham, R. E. and Brent, L.: Acquired tolerance of foreign cells in newborn animals. Proc. roy. Soc. B. 146: 78–90 (1956)

Billingham, R. E. and Brent, L.: Quantitative studies on tissue transplantation immunity. IV. Induction of tolerance in newborn mice and studies on the phenomenon of runt disease. Philos. Trans. (A/B) 242: 439–477 (1959).

Billingham, R. E.; Brent, L. and Medawar, P. B.: Actively acquired tolerance of foreign cells. Nature, Lond. 172: 603–605 (1953).

Billingham, R. E.; Brent, L. and Medawar, P. B.: Quantitative studies on tissue transplantation immunity. III. Actively acquired tolerance. Philos. Trans. (A/B) 239: 357–414 (1956 a).

Billingham, R. E.; Brent, L. and Medawar, P. B.: 'Enhancement' in normal homografts with a note on its possible mechanism. Transplant. Bull. 3: 84–88 (1956 b).

BILLINGHAM, R. E.; LAMPKIN, G. H.; MEDAWAR, P. B. and WILLIAMS, H. L.: Tolerance to homografts, twin diagnosis and the freemartin condition in cattle. Heredity 6: 201–212 (1952).

BILLINGHAM, R. E. and SILVERS, W. K.: The induction of tolerance of skin homografts in rats with pooled cells from multiple donors. J. Immunol. 83: 667–679 (1959).

BISHOP, D. W.: Aspermatogenesis induced by testicular antigen uncombined with adjuvant. Proc. Soc. exp. Biol., N. Y. 107: 116–120 (1961).

BLINKOFF, R. G.: γM and γG antibodies in mice: dissociation of the normal immunoglobulin sequence. J. Immunol. 97: 736–746 (1966).

BOLLAG, W.: Heterologe Transplantation von Tumoren bei Vorbehandlung der Empfängertiere mit Gewebe der Spendertiere während der Embryonalzeit. Experientia 11: 227 (1955).

BOOTH, P. B.; DUNSFORD, I.; GRANT, J. and MURRAY, S.: Haemolytic disease in first-born infants. Brit. med. J. ii: 41–42 (1953).

BOOTH, P. B.; PLAUT, G.; JAMES, J. D.; IKIN, E. W.; MOORES, P.; SANGER, R. and RACE, R. R.: Blood chimerism in a pair of twins. Brit. med. J. ii: 1456–1458 (1957).

BOREK, F.; STUPP, Y. and SELA, M.: Immunogenicity and role of size: response of guinea pigs to oligotyrosine and tyrosine derivatives. Science 150: 1177–1178 (1965).

BOREL, Y.; FAUCONNET, M. and MIESCHER, P. A.: Effect of 6-mercaptopurine (6-MP) on different classes of antibody. J. exp. Med. 122: 263–275 (1965).

BOREL, Y.; FAUCONNET, M. and MIESCHER, P. A.: Selective suppression of delayed hypersensitivity by the induction of immunologic tolerance. J. exp. Med. 123: 585–598 (1966).

BOYDEN, S. V.: The effect of previous injections of tuberculoprotein on the development of tuberculin sensitivity following BCG vaccination in guinea-pig. Brit. J. exp. Path. 38: 611–617 (1957).

BOYDEN, S. V. and SORKIN, E.: Effect of neonatal injections of protein on the immune response to protein-hapten complexes. Immunology 5: 370–377 (1962).

BRENT, L. and COURTENAY, T. H.: On the induction of split tolerance; in Mechanisms of Immunological Tolerance, p. 113 (Publ. House Czech. Acad. Sci., Prague 1962).

BRENT, L. and GOWLAND, G.: Cellular dose and age of host in the induction of tolerance. Nature, Lond. 192: 1265–1267 (1961).

BRENT, L. and GOWLAND, G.: Induction of tolerance of skin homografts in immunologically competent mice. Nature, Lond. 196: 1298–1301 (1962 a).

BRENT, L. and GOWLAND, G.: A quantitative analysis of tolerance induction in mice; in Mechanisms of Immunological Tolerance, p. 237 (Publ. House Czech. Acad. Sci., Prague 1962 b).

BRENT, L. and GOWLAND, G.: Immunological competence of newborn mice. Transplantation 1: 372–376 (1963).

BRENT, L. and MEDAWAR, P. B.: Quantitative studies on tissue transplantation immunity. V. The role of antiserum in enhancement and desensitization. Proc. roy. Soc. B. 155: 392–416 (1961).

BREYERE, E. J. and BARRETT, M. K.: 'Tolerance' in postpartum female mice induced by strain-specific matings. J. nat. Cancer Inst. 24: 699–705 (1960 a).

BREYERE, E. J. and BARRETT, M. K.: Prolonged survival of skin homografts in parous female mice. J. nat. Cancer Inst. 25: 1405–1410 (1960 b).

BREYERE, E. J. and BARRETT, M. K.: Tolerance induced by parity in mice incompatible at the H-2 locus. J. nat. Cancer Inst. 27: 409–417 (1961).

Brocades Zaalberg, O.; Vos, O. and Weyzen, W. W. H.: Influence of excess of antigen on immunological tolerance in radiation chimeras. Nature, Lond. *197:* 300–301 (1963).

Brooke, M. S.: Conversion of immunological paralysis to immunity by endotoxin. Nature, Lond. *206:* 635–636 (1965 a).

Brooke, M. S.: Decreased susceptibility to immunological paralysis with increased age. Transplantation *3:* 478–483 (1965 b).

Brooke, M. S. and Karnovsky, M. J.: Immunological paralysis and adoptive immunity. J. Immunol. *87:* 205–208 (1961).

Bubeník, J.; Iványi, J. and Koldovský, P.: Participation of 7 S and 19 S antibodies in enhancement and resistance to methylcholanthrene-induced tumours. Folia biol., Praha *11:* 426–433 (1965).

Burgio, G. R. e Severi, F.: Autoemoagglutinazione da liquido di bolla. Boll. Soc. ital. Biol. sper. *29:* 1987–1989 (1963).

Burgio, G. R. e Severi, F.: Ricerche sul liquido di bolla in rapporto a condizioni reattivo-allergiche locali. Riv. Clin. pediat. *73:* 72–89 (1964).

Burgio, G. R. und Severi, F.: Untersuchungen über Hämoagglutinine der Blasenflüssigkeit. Proc. 10th Congr. int. Soc. Blood Tranf., Stockholm 1964, p. 759 (Karger, Basel/New York 1965).

Burnet, F. M.: Enzyme, Antigen and Virus (Cambridge University Press, London 1956).

Burnet, F. M.: The Clonal Selection Theory of Acquired Immunity (Cambridge University Press, London 1959).

Burnet, F. M.: The immunological significance of the thymus: An extension of the clonal selection theory of immunity. Austr. Ann. Med. *11:* 79–91 (1962).

Burnet, M. F.: A Darwinian approach to immunity. Nature, Lond. *203:* 451–454 (1964).

Burnet, F. M. and Fenner, F.: The Production of Antibodies (Macmillan Co., Melbourne 1949).

Burnet, F. M. and Holmes, M. C.: Thymic changes in the mouse strain NZB in relation to the autoimmune state. J. Path. Bact. *88:* 229–241 (1964).

Burnet, F. M.; Stone, J. D. and Edney, M.: The failure of antibody production in the chick embryo. Austr. J. exp. Biol. med. Sci. *28:* 291–297 (1950).

Bussard, A.: Tolérance immunologique provoqué chez le lapin envers certains antigènes de la levure. C. R. Acad. Sci. *245:* 2430–2433 (1957).

Bussard, A. E.: Induction of immunological tolerance to yeast enzymes in mammals; in Mechanisms of Antibody Formation, p. 329 (Publ. House Czech. Acad. Sci., Prague 1960).

Bussard, A. E.: Immunological behaviour of rabbits towards human serum albumin two years after neonatal injection of the same antigen; in Mechanisms of Immunological Tolerance, p. 85 (Publ. House Czech. Acad. Sci., Prague 1962).

Bussard, A.: Définitions et critères de la tolérance immunologique; dans Tolérance acquise et la tolérance naturelle à l'égard de substances antigéniques définies, p. 9 (Centre National de la Recherche Scientifique, Paris 1963).

Bussard, A. and Huynh, V. A.: Incorporation of labelled amino-acids in antibodies synthesized *in vitro* by cells of immunized rabbits. Biochem. biophys. Res. Commun. *3:* 453–456 (1960).

Buxton, A.: Antibody production in avian embryos and young chicks. J. gen. Microbiol. *10:* 398–410 (1954).

Cannon, J. A. and Longmire, W. P.: Studies of successful skin homografts in the chicken. Ann. Surg. *135:* 60–68 (1952).

ČERNÝ, J. and IVÁNYI, J.: The dose of antigen required for the suppression of the IgM and IgG antibody response in chickens. II. Studies at the cellular level. Folia biol., Praha *12:* 343–354 (1966).

ČERNÝ, J.; IVÁNYI, J.; MADÁR, J. and HRABA, T.: The nature of the delay in the immune response after administration of large doses of protein antigen in chicks. Folia biol., Praha *11:* 402–405 (1965).

ČERNÝ, J. and VIKLICKÝ, V.: Effect of antigen dose on changes in the spleen: immunity versus tolerance? Exp. Hematology *11:* 28–29 (1966).

CHASE, M. W.: The cellular transfer of cutaneous hypersensitivity to tuberculin. Proc. Soc. exp. Biol., N. Y. *59:* 134–135 (1945).

CHASE, M. W.: Inhibition of experimental drug allergy by prior feeding of the sensitizing agent. Proc. Soc. exp. Biol., N. Y. *61:* 257–259 (1946).

CHASE, M. W.: Studies on the mechanism of inhibition of experimental drug allergy by prior feeding of the sensitizing agent. Abstr. 49th Gen. Meeting Soc. Amer. Bact., p. 75 (1949).

CHASE, M. W.: Experimental sensitization with particular reference to picryl chloride. Int. Arch. Allergy *5:* 163–191 (1954).

CHASE, M. W.: Immunological tolerance. Annu. Rev. Microbiol. *13:* 349–376 (1959).

CHASE, M. W.: Tolerance towards chemical allergens; dans Tolérance acquise et la tolérance naturelle à l'égard de substances antigéniques définies, p. 139 (Centre National de la Recherche Scientifique, Paris 1963).

CHOU, C.T.; DUBISKI, S. and CINADER, B.: Antibody formation and experimentally induced chimerism in very young rabbits. Nature, Lond. *211:* 34–36 (1966).

CHUTNÁ, J. and HRABA, T.: Attempt to induce immunological tolerance in rabbits by antigen (HSA)-antibody precipitate; in Mechanisms of Immunological Tolerance, p. 95 (Publ. House Czech. Acad. Sci., Prague 1962).

CHUTNÁ, J. and RYCHLÍKOVÁ, M.: Prevention and suppression of experimental autoimmune aspermatogenesis in adult guinea pigs. Folia biol., Praha *10:* 177–187 (1964 a).

CHUTNÁ, J. and RYCHLÍKOVÁ, M.: A study of the biological effectiveness of antibodies in the development and prevention of experimental autoimmune aspermatogenesis. Folia biol., Praha *10:* 188–197 (1964 b).

CHUTNÁ, J. and RYCHLÍKOVÁ, M.: Immunological tolerance to testicular antigen in immunized guinea pigs and the cytological changes in lymphoid organs. Folia biol., Praha *12:* 97–107 (1966).

CHUTNÁ, J.; VOJTÍŠKOVÁ, M.; RYCHLÍKOVÁ, M. and POKORNÁ, Z.: Attempt at the prevention of autoimmune aspermatogenesis; in Mechanisms of Immunological Tolerance, p. 511 (Publ. House Czech. Acad. Sci., Prague 1962).

CINADER, B.: Specificity and inheritance of antibody response: A possible steering mechanism. Nature, Lond. *188:* 619–622 (1960).

CINADER, B. and DUBERT, J. M.: Acquired immune tolerance to human albumin and the response to subsequent injections of diazoalbumin. Brit. J. exp. Path. *36:* 515–529 (1955).

CINADER, B. and DUBERT, J. M.: Specific inhibition of reponse to purified protein antigens. Proc. roy. Soc. B. *146:* 18–33 (1956).

CINADER, B. and DUBISKI, S.: The effect of immunogenicity of acquired immunological tolerance; dans Tolérance acquise et tolérance naturelle à l'égard de substances antigéniques définies, p. 255 (Centre National de la Recherche Scientifique, Paris 1963).

Cinader, B. and Dubiski, S.: Effect of autologous protein on the specificity of the anti-body response: mouse and rabbit antibody to MuB1. Nature, Lond. *202:* 102–103 (1964).

Cinader, B.: Dubiski, S. and Wardlaw, A. C.: Distribution, inheritance, and properties of an antigen, MuB1, and its relation to hemolytic complement. J. exp. Med. *120:* 897–924 (1964).

Cinader, B.; Dubiski, S. and Wardlaw, A. C.: Inheritance and properties of the antigen MuB1 and its relation to haemolytic complement. Nature, Lond. *205:* 97–98 (1965).

Cinader, B. and Pearce, J. H.: The specificity of acquired immunological tolerance to azo proteins. Brit. J. exp. Path. *39:* 8–29 (1958).

Cinader, B.; Pearce, J. H. and Carter, B. G.: Acquired immunological tolerance to bovine ribonuclease. Nature, Lond. *181:* 1208–1209 (1958).

Claman, H. N.: Tolerance to a protein antigen in adult mice and the effect of nonspecific factors. J. Immunol. *91:* 833–839 (1963).

Claman, H. N. and McDonald, W.: Thymus and x-radiation in the termination of acquired immunological tolerance in the adult mouse. Nature, Lond. *202:* 712–713 (1964).

Claman, H. N. and Talmage, D. W.: Thymectomy: prolongation of immunological tolerance in the adult mouse. Science *141:* 1193–1194 (1963).

Clarke, C. A.: Prevention of Rh haemolytic disease. A method based on the post-delivery injection of the mother with anti-D antibody. Vox Sang. *11:* 641–655 (1966).

Clarke, C. M.; Lengerová, A. and Micklem, H. S.: Futher observation on graft-versus-graft immunological tolerance in radiation chimaeras. Folia biol., Praha *8:* 335–340 (1962).

Coe, J. E. and Salvin, S. B.: The specificity of allergic reactions. VI. Unresponsiveness to simple chemicals. J. exp. Med. *117:* 401–423 (1963).

Cohen, M. W. and Thorbecke, G. J.: Interference by newborn lymphoid cells with establishment of immunologic unresponsiveness to protein antigens. Proc. Soc. exp. Biol., N. Y. *112:* 10–12 (1963).

Cohen, M. W. and Thorbecke, G. J.: Specificity of reaction of antigenic stimulation in lymph nodes of immature rabbits. II. Suppression of local morphology reaction to alum precipitated BSA by intraperitoneal injection of soluble BSA in neonatal rabbits. J. Immunol. *93:* 623–636 (1964).

Cohn, M.: The problem of specific inhibition of antibody synthesis in adult animals by immunization of embryos. Ann. N. Y. Acad. Sci. *64:* 859–876 (1957).

Cole, L. J. and Davis, W. E.: Specific homograft tolerance in lymphoid cells of long-lived radiation chimeras. Proc. nat. Acad. Sci., Wash. *47:* 594–602 (1961).

Collins, D. N.; Weigand, H. and Hotchin, J.: The effects of pretreatment with X-rays on the pathogenesis of lymphocytic choriomeningitis in mice. II. The pathological histology. J. Immunol. *87:* 682–687 (1961).

Coons, A. H.: Tolerance and persistence of antigen; dans Tolérance acquise et la tolérance naturelle à l'égard de substances antigéniques définies, p. 121 (Centre National de la Recherche Scientifique, Paris 1963).

Cotes, P. M.; Hobbs, K. R. and Bangham, D. R.: Development of the immune response in the foetal and newborn rhesus monkey. I. Response to bovine serum albumin. Immunology *11:* 185–198 (1966).

Crampton, C. F.; Frankel, F. R. and Rodeheaver, J. L.: Mechanism of immunological unresponsiveness. Nature, Lond. *184:* 873–875 (1959).

CROWLE, A. J.: Specific immunologic unresponsiveness to delayed hypersensitivity elicited in adult mice. Proc. Soc. exp. Biol., N. Y. *110:* 447–449 (1962).

CROWLE, A. J.: Immunologic unresponsiveness to protein antigens induced in adult hypersensitive mice. J. Allergy *34:* 504–519 (1963).

CURTAIN, C. C.: The use of acquired immunological tolerance and immunological 'paralysis' in the study of the antigenic relationships of normal and abnormal serum globulins. Brit. J. exp. Path. *40:* 255–262 (1959).

DACIE, J. V.: Hemolytic anemia. Ann. N. Y. Acad. Sci. *124:* 415–440 (1965).

DÉMANT, P.; IVÁNYI, P. and IVAŠKOVÁ, E.: Prolonged survival of maternal skin grafts in newborn rabbits. Ann. N. Y. Acad. Sci. *129/1:* 234–240 (1966).

DEMPSTER, W. J.: Kidney homotransplantation. Brit. J. Surg. *40:* 447–465 (1953).

DENHARDT, D. T. and OWEN, R. D.: The resistance of the tolerant state to irradiation. Transplant. Bull. *7:* 394–399 (1960).

DÉVÉNYI, I.; CZENKÁR, B. und ENDES, P.: Wirkung der Cortison-Adaptationsbehandlung auf das fetale und erwachsene Schilddrüsen- und Nebenschilddrüsen-Homoiotransplantat der Ratte. Frankf. Z. Path. *68:* 418–434 (1957a).

DÉVÉNYI, I.; CZENKÁR, B. und Endes, P.: Untersuchung der immunobiologischen Anpassung von Homoiotransplantaten. Frankf. Z. Path. *68:* 435–439 (1957 b).

DÉVÉNYI, I.; CZENKÁR, B. and ENDES, P.: Homotransplantation of adult rat thyroid and parathyroid with simultaneous cortisone treatment. Acta Morph. Acad Sci. Hung. *8:* 39–50 (1958 a).

DÉVÉNYI, I.; CZENKÁR, B. and ENDES, P.: Homotransplantation of foetal thyroid glands to temporarily cortisone-treated rats. Acta Morph. Acad. Sci. Hung. *8:* 59–69 (1958 b).

DÉVÉNYI, I.; CZENKÁR, B. and ENDES, P.: Relationship between cortisone dose and acquired tolerance in homotransplantation. Acta Morph. Acad. Sci. Hung. *8:* 139–144 (1958 c).

DÉVÉNYI, I.; CZENKÁR, B. and ENDES, P.: A study of the conditioning effect of non-continuous cortison treatment on the homografting of thyroid tissue in rats. Folia biol., Praha *8:* 230–232 (1962).

DÉVÉNYI, I.; KERTÉSZ, L. and CZENKÁR, B.: I^{131}-uptake of homotransplanted rat thyroids. Acta Biol. Acad. Sci. Hung. *8:* 325–331 (1958 d).

DE WECK, A. L. and FREY, J. R.: Immunotolerance to Simple Chemicals (Karger, Basel/New York 1966).

DIETRICH, F. M.: Relationship of antigenicity and degree of tolerance to heterologous serum albumins in C57 Bl/6 mice. Nature, Lond. *200:* 483 (1963).

DIETRICH, F. M. and GREY, H. M.: Quantity and quality of antibody produced following termination of tolerance in C57Bl/6 mice. Nature, Lond. *201:* 1236 (1964).

DIETRICH, F. M. and WEIGLE, W. O.: Induction of tolerance to heterologous proteins and their catabolism in C57Bl/6. J. exp. Med. *117:* 621–631 (1963)

DIETRICH, F. M. and WEIGLE, W. O.: Immunologic unresponsiveness to heterologous serum proteins induced in adult mice and transfer of the unresponsive state. J. Immunol. *92:* 167–172 (1964).

DIXON, F. J. and MAURER, P. H.: Immunological unresponsiveness induced by protein antigens. J. exp. Med. *101:* 245–257 (1955).

DIXON, F. J.; MAURER, P. H. and WEIGLE, W. O.: Immunologic activity of pneumococcal polysaccharide fixed in the tissues of the mouse. J. Immunol. *74:* 188–191 (1955).

DORNER, M. M. and UHR, J. W.: Immunologic tolerance after specific immunization. J. exp. Med. *120:* 435–447 (1964 a).

DORNER, M. M. and UHR, J. W.: The induction of immunological tolerance after specific antibody formation. Ann. N. Y. Acad. Sci. *120:* 424–429 (1964 b).

DOWDEN, S. J. and SERCARZ, E. E.: Spontaneous escape from BSA paralysis and its relationship to antigen contact. Fed. Proc. *25:* 488 (1966).

DOWNE, A. E. R.: Inhibition of the production of precipitating antibodies in young rabbits. Nature, Lond. *176:* 740–741 (1955).

DRESSER, D. W.: The effectiveness of lipid and lipidophilic substances as adjuvants. Nature, Lond. *191:* 1169–1171 (1961 a).

DRESSER, D. W.: Acquired immunological tolerance to a fraction of bovine γ-globulin. Immunology *4:* 13–23 (1961 b).

DRESSER, D.W.: Specific inhibition of antibody production. I. Protein-overloading paralysis. Immunology *5:* 161–168 (1962 a).

DRESSER, D. W.: Specific inhibition of antibody production. II. Paralysis induced in adult mice by small quantities of protein antigen. Immunology *5:* 378–388 (1962 b).

DRESSER, D. W.: Specific inhibition of antibody production. IV. Standardization of the antigen-elimination test; immunological paralysis of mice previously immunized. Immunology *9:* 261–273 (1965).

DRESSER, D. W. and GOWLAND, G.: Immunological paralysis induced in adult rabbits by small amounts of a protein antigen. Nature, Lond. *203:* 733–736 (1964).

DRESSER, D. W. and WORTIS, H. H.: Use of an antiglobulin serum to detect cells producing antibody with low haemolytic efficiency. Nature, Lond. *208:* 859–861 (1965).

DUBERT, J. E. et PARAF, A.: Etude quantitative des conditions nécessaires à l'apparition d'un état de tolérance immunitaire. C. R. Acad. Sci. *244:* 686 (1957).

DUNSFORD, I.; BOWLEY, C. C.; HUTCHISON, A. M.; THOMPSON, J. S.; SANGER, R. and RACE, R. R.: A human blood-group chimera. Brit. Med. J. *ii:* 81 (1953).

DUTTON, R. W.: The effect of antigen on the proliferation of spleen cell suspensions from tolerant rabbits. J. Immunol. *93:* 814–815 (1964).

DVORAK, H.; BILLOTE, J.; McCARTHY, J. and FLAX, M.: Immunologic unresponsiveness in the adult guinea pig. III. Variation of the antigen and vehicle of suppression. Induction of unresponsiveness in the adult rat. J. Immunol. *97:* 106–111 (1966).

DVORAK, H. F. and FLAX, M. H.: Immunologic unresponsiveness in the adult guinea pig. II. The kinetics of unresponsiveness. J. Immunol. *96:* 546–553 (1966).

FARR, R. S.: A quantitative immunochemical measure of the primary interaction between I^x B.S.A. and antibody. J. infect. Dis. *103:* 239–262 (1958).

FEFER, A. and DAVIS, W. C.: Induction of homograft tolerance in adult mice by sublethal x-irradiation and injection of homologous spleen cells. Transplantation *1:* 75–78 (1963).

FEFER, A. and NOSSAL, G. J. V.: Abolition of neonatally-induced homograft tolerance in mice by sublethal x-irradiation. Transplant. Bull. *29:* 445–451 (1962).

FELDMAN, M. and GLOBERSON, A.: Studies on the mechanism of immunological enhancement of tumor grafts. J. nat. Cancer Inst. *25:* 631–648 (1960).

FELDMAN, M.; GLOBERSON, A. and NACHTIGEL, D.: The reactivation of the immune response following x-irradiation and drug-induced immune tolerance; in Mechanisms of Immunological Tolerance, p. 305 (Publ. House Czech. Acad. Sci., Prague 1962).

FELDMAN, M. and YAFFE, D.: Immunogenetic studies on x-irradiated mice treated with homologous hematopoietic cells. J. nat. Cancer Inst. *21:* 697–712 (1958).

FELTON, L. D.: The significance of antigen in animal tissues. J. Immunol. *61:* 107–117 (1949).

FELTON, L. D.; KAUFFMANN, G.; PRESCOTT, B. and OTTINGER, B.: Studies on the mechanism of the immunological paralysis induced in mice by pneumococcal polysaccharides. J. Immunol. 74: 17–26 (1955 a).

FELTON, L. D. and OTTINGER, B.: Pneumococcus polysaccharides as a paralysing agent on the mechanism of immunity in white mice (abstract). J. Bact. 43: 94–95 (1942).

FELTON, L. D.; PRESCOTT, B.; KAUFFMANN, G. and OTTINGER, B.: Pneumococcal antigenic polysaccharide substances from animal tissues. J. Immunol. 74: 205–213 (1955 b).

FESTENSTEIN, H. and BOKKENHEUSER, V.: Attempted induction of immunological tolerance in rabbits using living Treponema pallidum. Brit. J. exp. Path. 42: 158–165 (1961).

FINKELSTEIN, M. S. and UHR, J. W.: Specific inhibition of antibody formation by passively administered 19S and 7S antibody. Science 146: 67–69 (1964).

FOLLETT, D. A.; BATTISTO, J. R. and BLOOM, B. R.: Tolerance to a defined chemical hapten produced in adult guinea pigs after thymectomy. Immunology 11: 73–76 (1966).

FREI, W.: Über willkürliche Sensibilisierung gegen chemisch definierte Substanzen. I. Mitteilung: Untersuchungen mit Neosalvarsan am Menschen. Klin. Wschr. 7: 539–542 (1928).

FREI, P. C.; BENACERRAF, B. and THORBECKE, G. J.: Phagocytosis of the antigen, a crucial step in the induction of the primary response. Proc. Nat. Acad. Sci., Wash. 53: 20–23 (1965).

FRENZL, B.; HAŠEK, M.; HAŠKOVÁ, V. and HRABA, T.: Immunological relationship in embryonic parabionts between duck and chicken I. (In Czech). Čs. biol. 4: 1–6 (1955).

FREY, J. R.; GELEICK, H. and DE WECK, A.: Immunological tolerance induced in animals previously sensitized to simple chemical compounds. Science 144: 853–854 (1964).

FRIEDMAN, H.: Prevention of immunologic unresponsiveness to Shigella antigens in neonatal mice by homologous spleen cell transplants. J. Immunol. 92: 201–207 (1964).

FRIEDMAN, H.: Failure of spleen cells from immunologically tolerant mice to form antibody plaques to sheep erythrocytes in agar gel. Nature, Lond. 205: 508–509 (1965 a).

FRIEDMAN, H.: Prevention of immunological tolerance to Shigella antigens in newborn mice by immune spleen cell extracts. Nature, Lond. 205: 1231–1232 (1965 b).

FRIEDMAN, H.: Prevention of immunologic tolerance by lymphoid cell transplants. Effect of time, cell concentration, injection route and type of cells transferred on establishment of unresponsiveness to Shigella antigens in neonatal mice. J. Immunol. 94: 205–213 (1965 c).

FRIEDMAN, H.: Adoptive tolerance to Shigella antigen in irradiated mice receiving spleen cell transplants from unresponsive donors. J. Immunol. 94: 352–357 (1965 d).

FRIEDMAN, H. and GABY, W. L.: Immunologic unresponsiveness to Shigella antigens in chickens. J. Immunol. 84: 441–448 (1960).

FUDENBERG, H. H. and FUDENBERG, B. R.: Antibody to hereditary human gamma-globulin (Gm) factor resulting from maternal-fetal incompatibility. Science 145: 170–171 (1964).

FUDENBERG, H. H.; GOODMAN, J. W. and MILGROM, F.: Immunochemical studies on rabbit anti-antibody. J. Immunol. 92: 227–233 (1964).

GALLILY, R. and FELDMAN, M.: Role of macrophages in the induction of antibody in x-irradiated animals. Exp. Hematology 11: 30 (1966).

GARVEY, J. S.; EITZMAN, D. V. and SMITH, R. T.: The distribution of S35-labeled bovine serum albumin in newborn and immunologically tolerant adult rabbits. J. exp. Med. 112: 533–550 (1960).

GENOVA, R. e VACCARO, R.: Contributo alla conoscenza della autoemoagglutinazione da liquido di bolla mediante il test dell'immunofluorescenza. Riv. Clin. pediat. *73:* 199–203 (1964).

GITLIN, D.; MÖNCKEGERG, F. and JANEWAY, C. A.: Effect of pneumococcus capsular polysaccharides on the degradation of rabbit antibodies in mice. J. Immunol. *86:* 627–634 (1961).

GOH, K.; MILLER, D. and DIAMOND, H. D.: An investigation into the use of 6-mercapto-purine to induce immunological tolerance. J. Immunol. *86:* 606–612 (1961).

GORMAN, J. G. and CHANDLER, J. G.: Is there immunologically incompetent lymphocyte? Blood *23:* 117–128 (1964).

GOŚCICKA, T.: Immunological unresponsiveness to streptococcal antigens. Bull. Acad. Pol. Sci. *11:* 23–28 (1963).

GOWLAND, G.: Induction of transplantation tolerance in adult animals. Brit. med. Bull. *21:* 123–128 (1965).

GOWLAND, G. and OAKLEY, C. L.: Acquired immunological tolerance of diphtheria alum-precipitated toxoid in the domestic fowl. J. Path. Bact. *80:* 373–378 (1960).

GREEN, I.; PAUL, W. E. and BENACERRAF, B.: The behavior of hapten-poly-l-lysine con-jugates as complete antigens in genetic responder and as haptens in nonresponder guinea-pigs. J. exp. Med. *123:* 859–879 (1966).

GREGG, M. B. and SALVIN, S. B.: Immunologic unresponsiveness to purified proteins in guinea pigs. J. Immunol. *90:* 368–371 (1963).

HAAS, V. H. and STEWART, S. E.: Sparing effect of a-methopterin and guanazolo in mice infected with the virus of lymphocytic choriomeningitis. Virology *2:* 511–516 (1956).

HALPERN, B. N.; LIACOPOULOS, P.; MARTIAL-LASFARGUES, C. et ARACTINGI, R.: Allonge-ment de la durée de survie des homogreffes cutanées chez le lapin et le cobaye au cours de la paralysie immunitaire induite par l'administration de γ-globulines hétérologues. C. R. Soc. Biol. *157:* 740–743 (1963).

HANAN, R. and OYAMA, J.: Inhibition of antibody formation in mature rabbits by contact with antigen at an early age. J. Immunol. *73:* 49–53 (1954).

HARRIS, T. N.; HARRIS, S. and FARBER, M. B.: Transfer of lymph node cells from rabbits injected with antigen. Fed. Proc. *11:* 470 (1952).

HARRIS, S.; HARRIS, T. N. and FARBER, M. B.: Studies on the transfer of lymph node cells. I. Appearance of antibody in recipients of cells from donor rabbits injected with antigen. J. Immunol. *72:* 148–160 (1954).

HAŠEK, M.: Parabiosis of birds during embryogenesis (in Czech). Čs. biol. *2:* 25–31 (1953a).

HAŠEK, M.: Vegetative hybridization of animals by joining their blood circulations during embryonic development (in Czech). Čs. biol. *2:* 265–277 (1953 b).

HAŠEK, M.: Manifestations of acquired tolerance in adaption of higher animals to foreign antigens (in Czech). Čs. biol. *3:* 327–332 (1954).

HAŠEK, M.: The problem of overcoming tissue incompatibility in homoplastic transfers (in Czech). Čas. lék. čes. *94:* 41–45 (1955).

HAŠEK, M.: Tolerance phenomena in birds. Proc. roy. Soc. B. *146:* 67–77 (1956).

HAŠEK, M.: Embryonic parabiosis and related problem of immunological tolerance. Transplant. Bull. *4:* 113–115 (1957).

HAŠEK, M.: Some problems of induction of transplantation tolerance; in Biological Pro-blems of Grafting, p. 1 (Université de Liège, 1959).

HAŠEK, M.: Immune tolerance to heterologous cells not capable of repopulation in the recipient. Folia biol., Praha *6:* 426–436 (1960).

Hašek, M.: Quantitative study of tolerance of skin grafts in ducks and the question of the adaption of grafts. Folia biol., Praha 7: 11–19 (1961).

Hašek, M.: Quantitative aspects of immunological tolerance. Folia biol., Praha 8: 73–83 (1962).

Hašek, M.: Introduction of immunologically competent cells into tolerant animals; dans Tolérance acquise et la tolérance naturelle à l'égaid de substances antigéniques définies, p. 217 (Centre National de la Recherche Scientifique, Paris 1963 a).

Hašek, M.: Critical factors governing the response pattern – immunity versus tolerance; in Immunopathology III, p. 148 (Schwabe & Co., Basel 1963 b).

Hašek, M.: Immunotoleranz; in Immunchemie, p. 268 (Springer, Berlin 1965 a).

Hašek, M.: Aspects cellulaires dans le développment de la tolérance immunitaire; dans Greffe et auto-immunité, p. 99 (Hermann, Paris 1965 b).

Hašek, M. and Hašková, V.: A contribution to the significance of individual antigenic specificity in homografting (in Czech). Čs. biol. 7: 282–283 (1958).

Hašek, M.; Hašková, V.; Lengerová, A. and Vojtíšková, M.: Mother-foetus immunological relationship as an exceptional homograft model; in: Ciba Foundation Symposium on Transplantation, p. 118 (Churchill, London 1962).

Hašek, M. and Hort, J.: Non-specific tolerance of graft and the dissociation of the two types of immunity. Nature, Lond. 186: 985–986 (1960).

Hašek, M. and Hort, J.: Variability of specificity in different models of tolerance; in Mechanisms of Immunological Tolerance, p. 143 (Publ. House Czech. Acad. Sci., Prague 1962).

Hašek, M.; Hort, J.; Lengerová, A. and Vojtíšková, M.: Immunological tolerance in the heterologous system. Folia biol., Praha 9: 1–9 (1963).

Hašek, M. and Hraba, T.: Immunological effects of experimental embryonal parabiosis. Nature, Lond. 175: 764–765 (1955 a).

Hašek, M. and Hraba, T.: The significance of phylogenetic kinship in immunological approximation during embryogenesis. Folia biol., Praha 1: 1–10 (1955 b).

Hašek, M.; Hraba, T. and Hort, J.: Embryonic parabiosis and related problems. Ann. N. Y. Acad. Sci. 73: 570–574 (1958).

Hašek, M.; Hraba, T. and Hort, J.: Acquired immunological tolerance of heterografts. Nature, Lond. 183: 1199–1200 (1959).

Hašek, M.; Hraba, T. and Hort, J.: Modification of immunological reactivity in turkey-chicken embryonic parabionts (Meleagris gallopavo L. and Gallus domesticus L.). Folia biol., Praha 6: 1–15 (1960).

Hašek, M.; Hraba, T. and Madar, J.: An attempt to characterize cellular background of partial tolerance. Folia biol., Praha 11: 318–320 (1965).

Hašek, M.; Hraba, T. and Madar, J.: The cellular background of partial tolerance; in Genetic Variations in Somatic Cells, p. 243 (Academia, Praha 1966a).

Hašek, M.; Iványi, J.; Bubeník, J. and Koldovský, P.: The significance of molecular characterization of serum antibodies in transplantation and tumor immunity. Ann. N. Y. Acad. Sci., 129, Art. 1: 787–792, (1966b).

Hašek, M.; Lengerová, A. and Hraba, T.: Transplantation immunity and tolerance; in: Adv. Immunology I, p. 1 (Academic Press, New York 1961).

Hašek, M. and Puza, A.: Induction of tolerance in adult life and reminiscence of tolerance; in Mechanisms of Immunological Tolerance, p. 257 (Publ. House Czech. Acad. Sci., Prague 1962 a).

Hašek, M. and Puza, A.: On the induction of immunological tolerance in adult recipients. Folia biol., Praha *8:* 55–57 (1962 b).

Hašek, M.; Svoboda, J. and Koldovský, P.: Immunological tolerance and the cancer problem. Acta Un. int. Cancer *19:* 102–104 (1963).

Hašková, V.: The adaptive period for foreign antigens in ontogenesis in ducks. Folia biol., Praha *3:* 129–134 (1957).

Hašková, V.: The relationship between the tissues of mother and foetus and tissue incompatibility. Folia biol., Praha *7:* 322–331 (1961).

Hašková, V.: Transplantation non-antigenicity of the foetal placenta. Nature, Lond. *193:* 278–279 (1962).

Hašková, V.: Differences in the antigenic effectiveness of the foetal part of mouse placenta depending on the strain combination employed. Folia biol., Praha *9:* 99–103 (1963).

Hašková, V. and Svoboda, J.: Relationship between transplantation immunity and immunological enhancement; in Mechanisms of Immunological Tolerance, p. 431 (Publ. House Czech. Acad. Sci., Prague 1962).

Hašková, V.; Svoboda, J. and Matoušek, V.: Relationship between transplantation immunity and immunological enhancement. Folia biol., Praha *8:* 16–20 (1962).

Hildemann, W. H. and Pinkerton, W.: Alloantibody production measured by plaque assay in relation to strong and weak histocompatibility. J. exp. Med. *124:* 885–900 (1966).

Hilgert, I.: Transplantation tolerance in adult mice induced with spleen cells and amethopterin. Folia biol., Praha *11:* 233–236 (1965).

Hirata, A. A.; Garvey, J. S. and Campbell, D. H.: Retention of antigen in tissues of serologically suppressed chickens. J. Immunol. *84:* 576–581 (1960).

Hirata, A. A. and Schechtman, A. M.: Studies on immunologic depression in chickens. J. Immunol. *85:* 230–239 (1960).

Holborow, E. J.; Asherson, G. L. and Wigley, R. D.: Auto-antibody production in rabbits. VI. The production of auto-antibodies against rabbit gastric, ileal and colonic mucosa. Immunology, Lond. *6:* 551–560 (1963).

Hort, J.; Hašek, M. and Knížetová, F.: Further immunological analysis of chicken embryonic parabionts, Folia biol., Praha *7:* 301–308 (1961).

Hotchin, J.: Latent infections of lymphocytic choriomeningitis virus; in Symposium on Latency and Masking in Viral and Rickettsial Infections, p. 59 (Burgess Pul. Co., Minneapolis 1958).

Hotchin, J. and Weigand, H.: Studies of lymphocytic choriomeningitis in mice. I. The relationship between age at inoculation and outcome of infection. J. Immunol. *86:* 392–400 (1961 a).

Hotchin, J. and Weigand, H.: The effects of pretreatment with x-rays on the pathogenesis of lymphocytic choriomeningitis in mice. I. Host survival, virus multiplication and leukocytosis. J. Immunol. *87:* 675–681 (1961 b).

Howard, J. G. and Michie, D.: Induction of transplantation immunity in the newborn mouse. Transplant. Bull. *29:* 91–96 (1962).

Hraba, T.: Immunological behaviour of embryonal parabionts between turkey and hen. Folia biol., Praha *2:* 165–171 (1956).

Hraba, T.: Immune tolerance to human serum in rabbits. Folia biol., Praha *5:* 312–316 (1959).

Hraba, T. and Hašek, M.: Skin homotransplants in day-old chicks, ducks and turkeys (in Russian). Folia biol., Praha *2:* 61–64 (1956).

HRABA, T.;HAŠEK, M. and ČUMLIVSKI, B.: Immunological approximation of sheep triplets, natural embryonic parabionts. Folia biol., Praha 2: 276–283 (1956).

HRABA, T. and IVÁNYI, J.: Comparison of tolerance to duck and human serum albumin in rabbits. Folia biol., Praha 9: 210–217 (1963).

HRABA, T.; MÁJSKÝ, A.; VÍTOVÁ, Z. and MATOUŠEK, V.: Influence of the mother's blood group on the formation of natural isoagglutinins by the child. Folia biol., Praha 8: 60–62 (1962).

HRABA, T. and MERCHANT, B.: Adaptation of the plaque technique for enumeration of cells producing antibody against a simple hapten. Fed. Proc. 25: 305 (1966).

HUMPHREY, J. H.: Acquired tolerance after treatment by physical or chemical agents; dans Tolérance acquise et tolérance naturelle à l'égard de substances antigéniques définies, p. 161 (Centre National de la Recherche Scientifique, Paris 1963).

HUMPHREY, J. H.: Immunological unresponsiveness to protein antigens in rabbits. I. The duration of unresponsiveness following a single injection at birth. Immunology, Lond. 7: 449–461 (1964 a).

HUMPHREY, J. H.: Immunological unresponsiveness to protein antigens in rabbits. II. The nature of the subsequent antibody response. Immunology, Lond. 7: 462–473 (1964 b).

HUMPHREY, J. H. and TURK, J. L.: Immunological unresponsiveness in guinea pigs. I. Immunological unresponsiveness to heterologous serum proteins. Immunology, Lond. 4: 301–309 (1961).

ILBERY, P. L. T.; KOLLER, P. C. and LOUTIT, J. F.: Immunological characteristics of radiation chimaeras. J. nat. Cancer Inst. 20: 1051–1090 (1958).

INGRAHAM, J. S. and BUSSARD, A.: Application of a localized hemolysin reaction for specific detection of individual antibody-forming cells. J. exp. Med. 119: 667–684 (1964).

ISACSON, P.: Cellular transfer of antibody production from adult to embryo in domestic fowls. Yale J. Biol. Med. 32: 209–228 (1959).

ISAKOVIĆ, K.; SMITH, S. B. and WAKSMAN, B. H.: Role of the thymus in tolerance. I. Tolerance to bovine γ-globulin in thymectomized, irradiated rats grafted with thymus from tolerant donors. J. exp. Med. 122: 1103–1123 (1965).

IVÁNYI, J. and ČERNÝ, J.: The effect of protein antigen dosage on its elimination from the blood and organs. Folia biol., Praha 11: 335–349 (1965).

IVÁNYI, J. and HRABA, T.: A contribution to the study of immunological tolerance to protein antigen in the chicken. Folia biol., Praha 9: 354–363 (1963).

IVÁNYI, J. and HRABA, T.: Characterization of antibodies in chicks after disappearance of immunological tolerance to human serum albumin. Folia biol., Praha 10: 409–411 (1964).

IVÁNYI, J.; HRABA, T. and ČERNÝ, J.: Immunological tolerance to human serum albumin (HSA) in chickens of adult and juvenile age. Folia biol., Praha 10: 198–205 (1964 a).

IVÁNYI, J.; HRABA, T. and ČERNÝ, J.: The elimination of heterologous and homologous serum proteins in chickens at various ages. Folia biol., Praha 10: 275–284 (1964 b).

IVÁNYI, J. and VALENTOVÁ, V.: The immunological significance of taxonomic origin of protein antigen in chickens. Folia biol., Praha 12: 36–48 (1966).

IVÁNYI, P.: Immunological tolerance in newborn rabbits. IV. Further studies on skin transplantation in newborn rabbits. Folia biol., Praha 10: 443–460 (1964).

IVÁNYI, P. and DÉMANT, P.: Prolonged survival of maternal skin grafts in newborn rabbits. Folia biol., Praha 11: 321–323 (1965).

Iványi, P. and Iványi, D.: The influence of the degree of relationship on the induction of tolerance in newborn rabbits; in Mechanisms of Immunological Tolerance, p. 165 (Publ. House Czech. Acad. Sci. Prague 1962).

Jakobowicz, R.; Crawford, H.; Graydon, J. J. and Pinder, M.: Immunological tolerance within the ABO blood group system. Brit. J. Haemat. *5:* 232–244 (1959).

Jerne, N. K. and Nordin, A. A.: Plaque formation in agar by single antibody-producing cells. Science *140:* 405 (1963).

Jerne, N. K.; Nordin, A. A. and Henry, C.: The agar plaque technique for recognizing antibody producing cells; in: Cell-Bound Antibodies, p. 109 (Wistar Inst. Press, Philadelphia 1963).

Johnson, A. G.; Watson, D. W. and Cromartie, W. J.: The effect of massive antigen dosage on antigen retention and antibody response in the rabbit. Proc. Soc. exp. Biol., N. Y. *88:* 421–427 (1955).

Johnston, G. D.; Asherson, G. L.; Kaklamanis, E. and Dumonde, D. C.: Demonstration by immunofluorescence of auto-antibody in the serum of rabbits given injections of rat tissue. J. Path. Bact. *86:* 521–525 (1963).

Jones, V. E. and Leskowitz, S.: Immunochemical study of antigenic specificity in delayed hypersensitivity. IV. The production of unresponsiveness to delayed hypersensitivity with a single antigenic determinant. J. exp. Med. *122:* 505–515 (1965).

Kaliss, N.: Course of production of an isoantiserum effecting tumor homograft survival in mice. Proc. nat. Acad. Sci., Wash. *42:* 269–273 (1956).

Kaliss, N.: Immunological enhancement of tumor homografts in mice. A review. Cancer Res. *18:* 992–1003 (1958).

Kaliss, N.: The induction of the homograft reaction in the presence of immunological enhancement of tumor homografts; in Mechanisms of Immunological Tolerance, p. 413 (Publ. House Czech. Acad. Sci., Prague 1962).

Kaliss, N. and Kandutsch, A.: Acceptance of tumor homografts by mice injected with antiserum. I. Activity of serum fractions. Proc. Soc. exp. Biol., N.Y. *91:* 118–121 (1956).

Kaliss, N.; Molomut, N.; Harris, J. L. and Gault, S. D.: Effect of previously injected immune serum and tissue on the survival of tumor grafts in mice. J. nat. Cancer Inst. *13:* 847–850 (1953).

Kantor, F. S.; Ojeda, A. and Benacerraf, B.: Studies on artificial antigens. I. Antigenicity of DNP-polylysine and DNP copolymers of lysine and glutamic acid in guinea pigs. J. exp. Med. *117:* 55–69 (1963).

Kaplan, M. H.: Immunologic studies of heart tissue. I. Production in rabbits of antibodies reactive with an autologous myocardial antigen following immunization with heterologous heart tissue. J. Immunol. *80:* 254–267 (1958).

Kaplan, M. H.: Immunologic relation of streptococcal and tissue antigens. I. Properties of an antigen in certain strains of group A streptococci exhibiting an immunologic cross-reaction with human heart tissue. J. Immunol. *90:* 595–606 (1963).

Kaplan, M. H. and Craig, J. M.: Immunologic studies of heart tissue. VI. Cardiac lesions in rabbits associated with autoantibodies to heart induced by immunization with heterologous heart. J. Immunol. *90:* 725–733 (1963).

Kaplan, M. H. and Suchy, M. L.: Immunologic relation of streptococcal and tissue antigens. II. Cross-reaction of antisera to mammalian heart tissue with a cell wall constitutent of certain strains of group A streptococci. J. exp. Med. *119:* 643–650 (1964).

Kaplan, M. H. and Svec, K. H.: Immunologic relation of streptococcal and tissue antigens. III. Presence in human sera of streptococcal antibody cross-reactive with heart tissue. Association with streptococcal infection, rheumatic fever, and glomerulone-phritis. J. exp. Med. *119:* 651–666 (1964).

KAPLAN, M. H.; COONS, A. H. and DEANE, H. W.: Localization of antigen in tissue cells. III. Cellular distribution of pneumococcal polysaccharides types II and III in the mouse. J. exp. Med. *91:* 15–30 (1950).

KATSH, S.: Localization and identification of antispermic factor in guinea pig testicles. Int. Arch. Allergy *16:* 241–275 (1960).

KERR, W. R. and ROBERTSON, M.: Passively and actively acquired antibodies. J. Hyg. *52:* 253–263 (1954).

KIES, M. W.: Panel discussion on species variability and multiple antigens in EAE: Summary statement. Ann. N. Y. Acad. Sci. *122:* 242–244 (1965).

KOLDOVSKÝ, P.: Homotransplantation in rats with polyvalent tolerance. Transplant. Bull. *28:* 119–121 (1961 a).

KOLDOVSKÝ, P.: Polyvalent tolerance to organ homografts in rats. Folia biol., Praha *7:* 98–102 (1961 b).

KOLDOVSKÝ, P.: Dangers and limitations of the immunological treatment of cancer. Lancet *i:* 654–655 (1966).

KOLDOVSKÝ, P.: Specific Antitumor Immunity (Springer-Verlag, Heidelberg, in press).

KOLDOVSKÝ, P. and SVOBODA, J.: Induction of tolerance to tumour antigen; in Mechanisms of Immunological Tolerance, p. 215 (Publ. House Czech. Acad. Sci., Prague 1962).

KOPROWSKI, H.: Actively acquired tolerance to a mouse tumor. Nature, Lond. *175:* 1087–1088 (1955).

KUNKEL, H. G. and TAN, E. M.: Autoantibodies and disease; in: Adv. Immunology IV, p. 351 (Academic Press, New York 1964).

LAMPKIN, G. H.: Intolerance of dizygotic twin lambs to skin homografts. Nature, Lond. *171:* 975–976 (1953).

LANDY, M.; SANDERSON, R. P. and JACKSON, A. L.: Humoral and cellular aspects of the immune response to the somatic antigen of Salmonella enteritidis. J. exp. Med. *122:* 483–504 (1965).

LEDERBERG, J.: Genes and antibodies. Science *129:* 1649–1653 (1959).

LEMMEL, E. M. and NOUZA, K.: Runt disease as a model of immunosuppressive therapy. Folia biol., Praha *12:* 253–265 (1966).

LENGEROVÁ, A.: Effect of irradiation during embryogenesis on the relationship between the maternal organism and offspring from the aspect of tissue compatibility. Folia biol., Praha *3:* 333–337 (1957).

LENGEROVÁ, A.: Concerning the problem of delayed death after transplantation of non-irradiated homologous tissue to lethally irradiated animals (in Czech.). Čs. biol. *7:* 285–286 (1958).

LENGEROVÁ, A.: Comparison of the therapeutic efficiency of homologous and heterologous embryonic haematopoietic cells administered to lethally irradiated mice. Folia biol., Praha *5:* 18–23 (1959).

LENGEROVÁ, A.: Polyvalent immunological tolerance in homologous radiation chimaeras. Nature, Lond. *187:* 160–161 (1960).

LENGEROVÁ, A.: The significance of immunological immaturity for the induction of toler-ance. J. theor. Biol. *3:* 503–508 (1962).

LENGEROVÁ, A.: Quantitative study on interactions of cellular grafts in mouse radiation chimaeras. Folia biol., Praha *9:* 196–202 (1963).

LENGEROVÁ, A. and MICKLEM, H. S.: Graft-versus-graft tolerance in radiation chimaeras; in Mechanisms of Immunological Tolerance, p. 379 (Publ. House Czech. Acad. Sci., Prague 1962).

LENGEROVÁ, A.; MICKLEM, H. S. and DENT, T.: Graft-versus-graft immunological tolerance in radiation chimaeras. Folia biol., Praha 7: 309–321 (1961).

LENGEROVÁ, A. and POLÁČKOVÁ, M.: The requirements for tolerance induction in cell-grafts from adult donors. Folia biol., Praha 9: 189–195 (1963).

LENGEROVÁ, A. and VOJTÍŠKOVÁ, M.: Postpartum reactivity of female mice to male specific antigens. Folia biol., Praha 8: 21–26 (1962).

LENGEROVÁ, A. and VOJTÍŠKOVÁ, M.: Prolonged survival of syngeneic male skin grafts in parous C57Bl mice. Folia biol., Praha 9: 72–74 (1963).

LENGEROVÁ, A. and VOJTÍŠKOVÁ, M.: Role of the thymus in mouse chimaeras. Folia biol., Praha 10: 245–249 (1964).

LESKOWITZ, S.: The use of antigen-antibody specific precipitates in skin testing for delayed hypersensitivity. J. Immunol. 85: 614–622 (1960).

LESKOWITZ, S.; JONES, V. E. and ZAK, S. J.: Immunochemical study of antigenic specificity in delayed hypersensitivity. V. Immunization with monovalent low molecule weight conjugates. J. exp. Med. 123: 229–237 (1966).

LEVINE, B. B. and BENACERRAF, B.: Genetic control in guinea pigs of the immune response to conjugates of haptens and poly-l-lysine. Science 147: 517–518 (1964 a).

LEVINE, B. B. and BENACERRAF, B.: Studies on antigenicity. The relationship between in vivo and in vitro enzymatic degradability of hapten-polylysine conjugates and their antigenicities in guinea pigs. J. exp. Med. 120: 955–965 (1964 b).

LEVINE, B. B.; OJEDA, A. and BENACERRAF, B.: Basis for the antigenicity of hapten-poly-l-lysine conjugates in random-bred guinea pigs. Nature, Lond. 200: 544–546 (1963 a).

LEVINE, B. B.; OJEDA, A. and BENACERRAF, B.: Studies on artificial antigens. III. The genetic control of the immune response to hapten poly-l-lysine conjugates in guinea pigs. J. exp. Med. 118: 953–957 (1963 b).

LIACOPOULOS, P.: Inhibition des réponses immunologiques après administration de doses élévées d'une protéine hétérologue. C. R. Acad. Sci. 253: 751–753 (1961).

LIACOPOULOS, P.: Suppression of immunological responses during the induction of immune paralysis with unrelated antigens. Texas Rep. Biol. Med. 23: 63–80 (1965).

LIACOPOULOS, P. and GOODE, J. H.: Transplantation tolerance induced in adult mice by protein overloading of donors. Science 146: 1305–1307 (1964).

LIACOPOULOS, P.; HALPERN, B. N. and PERRAMANT, F.: Unresponsiveness to unrelated antigens induced by paralysing doses of bovine serum albumin. Nature, Lond. 195: 1112–1113 (1962).

LIACOPOULOS, P. and NEVEU, TH.: Non-specific inhibition of the immediate and delayed types of hypersensitivity during immune paralysis of adult guinea-pigs. Immunology, Lond. 7: 26–39 (1964).

LIACOPOULOS, P. et STIFFEL, C.: Inhibition de la maladie homologue chez des souris hybrides F₁ adultes par un traitement des animaux donneurs et receveurs avec des γ-globulines de lapin. Rev. franç. Et. clin. biol. 8: 587–591 (1963).

LINSCOTT, W. D. and WEIGLE, W. O.: Anti-B.S.A. specificity and binding affinity after termination of tolerance to B.S.A. J. Immunol. 95: 546–558 (1965).

LOEWI, G.; HOLBOROW, E. J. and TEMPLE, A.: Inhibition of delayed hypersensitivity by pre-immunization without complete adjuvant. Immunology, Lond. 10: 339–347 (1966).

MAGUIRE, H. C. and MAIBACH, H. I.: Specific immune tolerance to anaphylactic sensitization (egg albumin) induced in the guinea pig by cyclophosphoramide (Cytoxan). J. Allergy *32:* 406–408 (1961).

MÄKELÄ, O. and MITCHISON, N. A.: The role of cell number and source in adoptive immunity. Immunology, Lond. *8:* 539–548 (1965 a).

MÄKELÄ, O. and MITCHISON, N. A.: The effect of antigen dosage on the response of adoptively transferred cells. Immunology, Lond. *8:* 549–556 (1965 b).

MÄKELÄ, O. and NOSSAL, G. J. V.: Accelerated breakdown of immunological tolerance following whole body irradiation. J. Immunol. *88:* 613–620 (1962).

MAKINODAN, T.; HOPPER, I.; SADO, T. and CAPALBO, E.: The suppressive effect of supra-optimal dose of antigen on the secondary antibody-forming response of spleen cells cultured in cell-impermeable diffusion chambers. J. Immunol. *95:* 466–479 (1965).

MARIANI, T.; MARTINEZ, C.; SMITH, J. M. and GOOD, R. A.: Induction of immunological tolerance to male skin isografts in female mice subsequent to neonatal period. Proc. Soc. exp. Biol., N. Y. *101:* 596–599 (1959).

MARK, R. and DIXON, F. J.: Anti-bovine serum albumin formation by transferred hyperimmune mouse spleen cells. J. Immunol. *91:* 614–620 (1963).

MARTIN, W. J.: The cellular basis of immunological tolerance in newborn animals. Austr. J. exp. Biol. med. Sci. *44:* 605–608 (1966).

MARTINEZ, C.; SHAPIRO, F. and GOOD, R. A.: Induction of immunological tolerance of tissue homografts in adult mice; in Mechanisms of Immunological Tolerance, p. 329 (Publ. House Czech. Acad. Sci., Prague 1962).

MARTINEZ, C.; SMITH, J. M.; BLAESE, M. and GOOD, R. A.: Production of immunological tolerance in mice after repeated injections of disrupted spleen cells. J. exp. Med. *118:* 743–758 (1963).

MATHÉ, G.; BINET, J. L.; SEMAN, G.; AMIEL, J. L. et DAGUET, G.: Cellules immunologiquement compétentes, immunité et tolérance; dans Tolérance acquise et tolérance naturelle à l'égard de substances antigéniques définies, p. 359 (Centre National de la Recherche Scientifique, Paris 1963).

MAYEDA, K.: Study of tolerance to the ABO blood group antigens. Vox Sang. *11:* 33–37 (1966).

McBRIDE, R. A. and SCHIERMAN, L. W.: Antibody-forming cells: population patterns after simultaneous immunization with different isoantigens. Science *154:* 655–657 (1966).

McCLUSKEY, R. T.; MILLER, F. and BENACERRAF, B.: Sensitization to denaturer autologous γ-globulin. J. exp. Med. *115:* 253–273 (1962).

McDEVITT, H. O. and SELA, M.: Genetic control of the antibody response. I. Demonstration of determinant specific differences in response to synthetic polypeptide antigens in two strains of inbred mice. J. exp. Med. *122:* 517–531 (1965).

McKHANN, C. F.: Weak histocompatibility genes: the effect of dose and pretreatment of immunizing cells. J. Immunol. *88:* 500–504 (1962).

McLAREN, A.: Induction of tolerance to skin homografts in adult mice treated with 6-mercaptopurine. Transplant. Bull. *28:* 479–484 (1961).

MEDAWAR, P. B.: Immunity to homologous grafted skin. II. The relationship between the antigens of blood and skin. Brit. J. exp. Path. *27:* 15–24 (1946).

MEDAWAR, P. B.: Introduction; in Mechanisms of Immunological Tolerance, p. 17 (Publ. House Czech. Acad. Sci., Prague (1962).

MEDAWAR, P. B.: The use of antigenic tissue extracts to weaken the immunological reaction against skin homografts in mice. Transplantation *1:* 21–38 (1963).

MERCHANT, B. and HRABA, T.: Lymphoid cells producing antibody against simple haptens: detection and enumeration. Science, *152:* 1378–1379 (1966).

MERCHANT, B.; HRABA, T. and HARRELL, B.: Immunological tolerance to sulfanilic acid assessed by the hemolytic plaque technique. Fed. Proc. *26:* 751 (1967).

MEYER, R. K.; ASPINALL, R. L.; GRAETZER, M. A. and WOLFE, H. R.: Effect of cortico-sterone on the skin homograft reaction and on precipitin and hemagglutinin production in thymectomized and bursectomized chickens. J. Immunol. *92:* 446–451 (1964).

MICHIE, D. and WOODRUFF, M. F. A.: Induction of specific immunological tolerance of homografts in adult mice by sublethal irradiation and injection of donor-type spleen cells in high dosage. Proc. roy. Soc. B. *156:* 280–288 (1962).

MICHIE, D.; WOODRUFF, M. F. A. and ZEISS, I. M.: An investigation of immunological tolerance based on chimaera analysis. Immunology, Lond. *4:* 413–424 (1961).

MICKLEM, H. S. and LOUTIT, J. F.: Tissue Grafting and Radiation (Academic Press, New York 1966).

MILGROM, F.: Rabbit sera with 'anti-antibody'. Vox Sang. *7:* 545–558 (1962).

MILGROM, F.; DUBISKI, S. and WOZNICZKO, G.: A simple method of Rh determination. Nature, Lond. *178:* 539 (1956 a).

MILGROM, F.; DUBISKI, S. and WOZNICZKO, G.: Human sera with 'anti-antibody'. Vox Sang. *1:* 172–183 (1956 b).

MILGROM, F. and WITEBSKY, E.: Studies on the rheumatoid and related serum factors. J. amer. med. Ass. *174:* 56–63 (1960).

MILGROM, F.; WICHER, K. and ROGALA, D.: Effect of intra-embryonic injections of BCG on the survival time in the tuberculous guinea pig. Schweiz. Z. Path. Bakt. *21:* 89–92 (1958).

MILGROM, F.; WOZNICZKO, G. and DUDZIAK, Z.: Physiological production of auto-antibodies. Schweiz. Z. Path. Bakt. *20:* 373–381 (1957).

MITCHELL, J. and NOSSAL, G. J. V.: Mechanism of induction of immunological tolerance. I. Localization of tolerance-inducing antigen. Austr. J. exp. Biol. med. Sci. *44:* 211–224 (1966).

MITCHISON, N. A.: Passive transfer of transplantation immunity. Nature, Lond. *171:* 267–268 (1953).

MITCHISON, N. A.: Passive transfer of transplantation immunity. Proc. roy. Soc. B. *142:* 72–87 (1954).

MITCHISON, N. A.: Blood transfusion in fowl: an example of immunological tolerance requiring the persistence of antigen; in Biological Problems of Grafting, p. 239 (Université de Liège, 1959).

MITCHISON, N. A.: Tolerance of erythrocytes in poultry: Induction and specificity. Immunology, Lond. *5:* 341–358 (1962 a).

MITCHISON, N. A.: Tolerance of erythrocytes in poultry: Loss and abolition. Immunology, Lond. *5:* 359–369 (1962 b).

MITCHISON, N. A.: Long-term processes in paralysis; in Mechanisms of Immunological Tolerance, p. 245 (Publ. House Czech. Acad. Sci., Prague 1962 c).

MITCHISON, N. A.: Induction of immunological paralysis in two zones of dosage. Proc. roy. Soc. B. *161:* 275–292 (1964).

MITCHISON, N. A.: Recovery from immunological paralysis in relation to age and residual antigen. Immunology, Lond. *9:* 129–138 (1965).

MITCHISON, N. A.: Recognition of antigen by cells. Progr. Biophys. Molecul. Biol. *16:* 3–14 (1966).

MÖLLER, G.: Studies on the mechanism of immunological enhancement of tumor homografts. I. Specificity of immunological enhancement. J. nat. Cancer Inst. *30:* 1153–1175 (1963 a).

MÖLLER, G.: Studies on the mechanism of immunological enhancement of tumor homografts. II. Effect of isoantibodies on various tumor cells. J. nat. Cancer Inst. *30:* 1177–1203 (1963 b).

MÖLLER, G.: Studies on the mechanism of immunological enhancement of tumor homografts. III. Interaction between humoral isoantibodies and immune lymphoid cells. J. nat. Cancer Inst. *30:* 1205–1226 (1963 c).

MÖLLER, G.: Prolonged survival of allogeneic (homologous) normal tissues in antiserum-treated recipients. Transplantation *2:* 281–286 (1964 a).

MÖLLER, G.: Antibody-induced depression of the immune response: a study of the mechanism in various immunological systems. Transplantation *2:* 405–415 (1964 b).

MÖLLER, G. and WIGZELL, H.: Antibody synthesis at the cellular level. Antibody-induced suppression of 19S and 7S antibody response. J. exp. Med. *121:* 969–989 (1965).

MOORE, N. W. and ROWSON, L. E. A.: Freemartins in sheep. Nature, Lond. *182:* 1754 to 1755 (1958).

MUELLER, A. P.: Prolonged antibody production following attempts to induce immune unresponsiveness in adult and juvenile chickens. Folia biol., Praha *13:* 18–28 (1967).

MUELLER, A. P. and WOLFE, H. R.: Precipitin production following massive injection of BSA in adult chickens. Int. Arch. Allergy *19:* 321–330 (1961).

NACHTIGAL, D. and FELDMAN, M.: Immunological unresponsiveness to protein antigens in rabbits exposed to x-irradiation or 6-mercaptopurine treatment. Immunology, Lond. *6:* 356–369 (1963).

NACHTIGAL, D. and FELDMAN, M.: The immune response to azo-protein conjugates in rabbits unresponsive to the protein carriers. Immunology, Lond. *7:* 616–625 (1964).

NAGY, L. K.: The effect of Brucella infection of young lambs on their serological responsiveness to the same antigens later in life. Immunology, Lond. *6:* 48–63 (1963).

NAKIĆ, B. and SILOBRČIĆ, V.: Specificity of tolerance following shortterm parabiosis between immunologically mature albino rats; in Mechanism of Immunological Tolerance, p. 337 (Publ. House Czech. Acad. Sci., Prague 1962).

NATHAN, H. C.; BIEBER, S.; ELION, G. B. and HITCHINGS, G. K.: Detection of agents which interfere with the immune response. Proc. Soc. exp. Biol., N. Y. *107:* 796–799 (1961).

NEEPER, C. A.: Mechanisms of immunologic paralysis by pneumococcal polysaccharide. III. Immunologic paralysis in relation to maturation of the immunologic response of mice. J. Immunol. *93:* 860–871 (1964).

NEEPER, C. A. and SEASTONE, C. V.: Mechanisms of immunologic paralysis by pneumococcal polysaccharide. I. Studies on adoptively acquired immunity to pneumococcal infection in immunologically paralyzed and normal mice. J. Immunol. *91:* 374–383 (1963).

NEIDERS, M. E.; ROWLEY, D. A. and FITCH, F. W.: The sustained suppression of hemolysin response in passively immunized rats. J. Immunol. *88:* 718–724 (1962).

NELSON, D. S.: Immunological enhancement of skin homografts in guinea pigs. Brit. J. exp. Path. *43:* 1–11 (1962).

NEVEU, TH.: Etude de la compétition des antigènes chez le cobaye adulte. Effect sur l'induction de l'hypersensibilité retardée et sur la formation d'anticorps envers une protéine homologue conjugée avec le chlorure de picryle. Ann. Inst. Pasteur *107:* 320–339 (1964).

NEVEU, T.; HALPERN, B. N.; LIACOPOULOS, P.; BIOZZI, G. and BRANELLEC, A.: Repression of delayed hypersensitivity to conjugated serum albumin during immune paralysis induced in guinea pig by heterologous proteins. Nature, Lond. *197:* 1023–1024 (1963).

NICHOLAS, J. W.; JENKINS, W. J. and MARSH, W. L.: Human blood chimeras. A study of surviving twins. Brit. med. J. *i:* 1458 (1957).

NISONOFF, A.; MARGOLIASH, E. and REICHLIN, M.: Antibodies to rabbit cytochrome c arising in rabbits. Science *155:* 1273–1275 (1967).

NOSSAL, G. J. V.: The immunological response of foetal mice to influenza virus. Austr. J. exp. Biol. med. Sci. *35:* 549–558 (1957).

NOSSAL, G. J. V.: Immunological tolerance: A new model system for low zone induction. Ann. N. Y. Acad. Sci. *129:, art. 1* 822–833 (1966).

NOSSAL, G. J. V. and ADA, G. L.: Recognition of foreignness in immune and tolerant animals. Nature, Lond. *201:* 580–582 (1964).

NOSSAL, G. J.V.; ADA, G. L. and AUSTIN, C. M.: Antigens in immunity. X. Induction of immunological tolerance to Salmonella adelaide flagellin. J. Immunol. *95:* 665–672 (1965).

NOSSAL, G. J. V. and AUSTIN, C. M.: Mechanism of induction of immunological tolerance. II. Simultaneous development of priming and tolerance. Austr. J. exp. Biol. med. Sci. *44:* 327–340 (1966).

NOSSAL, G. J. V.; FEFER, A. and MÄKELÄ, O.: Tolerance and irradiation; in Mechanisms of Immunological Tolerance, p. 151 (Publ. House Czech. Acad. Sci., Prague 1962).

NOSSAL, G. J. V. and MÄKELÄ, O.: Inhibition and restoration of specific immune responses; in Immunochemical Approaches to Problems in Microbiology, p. 377 (Institue of Microbiology, Rutgers, The State University, New Brunswick 1961).

OUDIN, J.: The genetic control of immunoglobulin synthesis. Proc. roy. Soc. B. *166:* 207–219 (1966).

OVARY, Z. and SPIEGELMAN, J.: The production of cold 'autohemagglutinins' in the rabbit as a consequence of immunization with isologous erythrocytes. Ann. N. Y. Acad. Sci. *124:* 147–153 (1965).

OWEN, R. D.: Immunogenetic consequences of vascular anastomoses between bovine twins. Science *102:* 400–402 (1945).

OWEN, R. D.: Erythrocyte antigens and tolerance phenomena. Proc. roy. Soc. B. *146:* 8–18 (1956).

OWEN, R. D.; WOOD, H. R.; FORD, A. G.; STURGEON, P. and BALDWIN, L. G.: Evidence for actively acquired tolerance to Rh antigens. Proc. nat. Acad. Sci., Wash. *40:* 420–424 (1954).

PARAF, A.; FOUGEREAU, M. et BUSSARD, A.: Rôle de l'adjuvant de Freund dans l'induction de la tolérance immunitaire à l'albumine humaine; dans Tolérance acquise et la tolérance naturelle à l'égard de substances antigéniques définies, p. 97 (Centre National de la Recherche Scientifique, Paris 1963).

PATERSON, P. Y.: Studies of immunological tolerance to nervous tissue in rats. Ann. N. Y. Acad. Sci. *73:* 811–817 (1958).

PATERSON, P. Y.: Transfer of allergic encephalomyelitis in rats by means of lymph node cells. J. exp. Med. *111:* 119–136 (1960).

PATERSON, P. Y. and HARWIN, S. M.: Suppression of allergic encephalomyelitis by means of immune serum; in Mechanisms of Immunological Tolerance, p. 507 (Publ. House Czech. Acad. Sci., Prague 1962).

PATERSON, P. Y. and HARWIN, S. M.: Suppression of allergic encephalomyelitis in rats by means of antibrain serum. J. exp. Med. *117:* 755–774 (1963).

PATERSON, P. Y.; HARWIN, S. M. and DIDAKOW, N. C.: Acquired resistance to allergic encephalomyelitis and the role of a serum factor. J. clin. Invest. 40: 1069–1070 (1961).

PERLMANN, P.; HAMMARSTRÖM, S.; LAGERCRANTZ, R. and GUSTAFSSON, B. E.: Antigen from colon of germfree rats and antibodies in human ulcerative colitis. Ann. N. Y. Acad. Sci. 124: 377–394 (1965).

PINCHUCK, P. and MAURER, P. H.: Antigenicity of polypeptides (poly alpha amino acids). XVI. Genetic control of immunogenicity of synthetic polypeptides in mice. J. exp. Med. 122: 673–679 (1965).

POKORNÁ, Z. and VOJTÍŠKOVÁ, M.: Autoimmune damage of the testes induced with chemically modified organ specific antigen. Folia biol., Praha 10: 261–267 (1964 a).

POKORNÁ, Z. and VOJTÍŠKOVÁ, M.: Ontogenic manifestation of the testicular antigen and the inducibility of autoimmune lesion by means of immature guinea pig testes. Folia biol., Praha 10: 392–398 (1964 b).

POKORNÁ, Z. and VOJTÍŠKOVÁ, M.: Reduced inducibility of autoimmune condition by passive transfer of immune and normal sera. Folia biol., Praha 10: 405–408 (1964 c).

POKORNÁ, Z. and VOJTÍŠKOVÁ, M.: Nonspecific inhibition of various types of immune response by means of normal serum. Folia biol., Praha 12: 88–96 (1966).

PORTER, K. A.: Runt disease and tolerance in rabbits. Nature, Lond. 185: 789–790 (1960).

PREHN, R. T.: Specific homograft tolerance induced by successive matings and implications concerning choriocarcinoma. J. nat. Cancer Inst. 25: 883–886 (1960).

PREHN, R. T. and THURSH, D. R.: The immunologic status of long-term radiation induced chimeras; in Mechanisms of Immunological Tolerance, p. 397 (Publ. House Czech. Acad. Sci., Prague 1962).

RAJEWSKY, K.: Rabbit antibody to pig lactic dehydrogenase reacting with the rabbit's own enzyme. Immunochemistry 3: 487–489 (1966).

RAPACZ, J.; SHACKELFORD, R. M. and JAKÓBIEC, J.: Blood groups studies in the domestic mink; in: Blood Groups of Animals, p. 211 (Publ. House Czech. Acad. Sci., Prague 1965).

REES, R. J.W. and GARBUTT, E. W.: Development of immunity to tuberculosis in adult mice injected with tubercle bacilli during foetal life. Immunology, Lond. 4: 88–93 (1961).

ROITT, I. M. and DONIACH, D.: Delayed hypersensitivity in auto-immune disease. Brit. med. Bull. 23: 66–71 (1967).

ROSE, N. R.; METZGAR, R. S. and WITEBSKY, E.: Studies on organ specificity. XI. Isoantigens of rabbit pancreas. J. Immunol. 85: 575–587 (1960).

ROWE, W. P.: Protective effect of preirradiation on lymphocytic choriomeningitis infection in mice. Proc. Soc. exp. Biol., N. Y. 92: 194–198 (1956).

ROWLEY, D. A. and FITCH, F. W.: Homeostasis of antibody formation in the adult rat. J. exp. Med. 120: 987–1005 (1964).

ROWLEY, D. A. and FITCH, F. W.: The mechanism of tolerance produced in rats to sheep erythrocytes. J. exp. Med. 121: 671–681 (1965 a).

ROWLEY, D. A. and FITCH, F. W.: The mechanism of tolerance produced in rats to sheep erythrocytes. II. The plaque-forming cell and antibody response to multiple injections of antigen begun at birth. J. exp. Med. 121: 683–695 (1965 b).

RYCHLÍKOVÁ, M. and CHUTNÁ, J.: Polyvalent tolerance in newborn and sublethally irradiated adult mice. Folia biol., Praha 11: 187–193 (1965).

SAHIAR, K. and SCHWARTZ, R. S.: Inhibition of 19S antibody synthesis by 7S antibody. Science 145: 395–397 (1964).

SAHIAR, K. and SCHWARTZ, R. S.: The immunoglobulin sequence. I. Arrest by 6-mercap-topurine and restitution by antibody, antigen or splenectomy. J. Immunol. *95:* 345–354 (1965).

SALVIN, S. B. and SMITH, R. F.: The specificity of allergic reactions. VII. Immunologic unresponsiveness, delayed hypersensitivity and circulating antibody to proteins and hapten protein conjugates in adult guinea pigs. J. exp. Med. *119:* 851–868 (1964).

SANDER, I. und STICHNOTH, A.: Gm-Antikörper bei Kleinkindern. Blut *9:* 102–103 (1963).

SANG, J. H. and SOBEY, W. R.: The genetic control of response to antigenic stimuli. J. Immunol. *72:* 52–65 (1954).

SCHECHTER, I.; BAUMINGER, S.; SELA, M.; NACHTIGAL, D. and FELDMAN, M.: Immune response to polypeptidyl proteins in rabbits tolerant to the protein carriers. Immunochemistry *1:* 249–265 (1964).

SCHINKEL, P. G. and FERGUSON, K. A.: Skin transplantation in the foetal lamb. Austr. J. Biol. Sci. *6:* 533–546 (1953).

SCHWARTZ, R. and DAMESHEK, W.: Drug induced immunological tolerance. Nature, Lond. *183:* 1682–1683 (1959).

SCHWARTZ, R. S. and DAMESHEK, W.: The role of antigen dosage in drug-induced immunologic tolerance. J. Immunol. *90:* 703–710 (1963).

SERCARZ, E. and COONS, A. H.: Specific inhibition of antibody formation during immunological paralysis and unresponsiveness. Nature, Lond. *184:* 1080–1082 (1959).

SERCARZ, E. and COONS, A. H.: The absence of antibody producing cells during unresponsiveness to BSA in the mice. J. Immunol. *90:* 478–491 (1963).

SERCARZ, E.; IVÁNYI, J. and POKORNÁ, Z.: Effect of antigen on the actinomycin-D sensitivity of the immune response in chicken spleen cultures. Fed. Proc. *26:* 751 (1967).

SHAPIRO, F.; MARTINEZ, C.; SMITH, J. M. and GOOD, R. A.: Tolerance of skin homografts induced in adult mice by multiple injections of homologous spleen cells. Proc. Soc. exp. Biol., N. Y. *106:* 472–475 (1961).

SIMMONS, R. L. and RUSSELL, P. S.: The antigenicity of mouse trophoblast. Ann. N. Y. Acad. Sci. *99:* 717–732 (1962).

SIMONSEN, M.: Biological incompatibility in kidney transplantation in dogs. II. Serological investigations. Acta path. microbiol. scand. *32:* 36–84 (1953).

SIMONSEN, M.: Induced tolerance to heterologous cells and induced susceptibility to virus. Nature, Lond. *175:* 763–764 (1955).

SISKIND, G. W. and HOWARD, J. G.: Studies on the induction of immunological unresponsiveness to pneumococcal polysaccharide in mice. J. exp. Med. *124:* 417–429 (1966).

SISKIND, G. W. and PATERSON, P. Y.: A bioassay for estimation of pneumococcal polysaccharide in unresponsive (paralyzed) mice. J. Immunol. *93:* 489–494 (1964).

SISKIND, G. W.; PATERSON, P. Y. and THOMAS, L.: Induction of unresponsiveness and immunity in newborn and adult mice with pneumococcal polysaccharide. J. Immunol. *90:* 929–934 (1963).

SKOWRON-CENDRZAK, A.: Phenomenon of parabiotic neutralization in mice; in Mechanisms of Immunological Tolerance, p. 323 (Publ. House Czech. Acad. Sci., Prague 1962).

SKOWRON-CENDRZAK, A.: Facilitation of homograft tolerance in parabiotic mice by treatment with amethopterin. Transplantation *2:* 487–495 (1964).

SLEE, J.: Immunological tolerance between littermates in sheep. Nature, Lond. *200:* 654–656 (1963).

SMITH, R. T.: Studies on the mechanism of immune tolerance; in Mechanisms of Antibody Formation, p. 313 (Publ. House Czech. Acad. Sci., Prague 1960).

SMITH, R. T.: Immunological tolerance of non-living antigens; in Adv. Immunology I, p. 67 (Academic Press, New York 1961).

SMITH, R. T. and BRIDGES, R. A.: Response of rabbits to defined antigens following neo-natal injection. Transplant. Bull. 3: 145–147 (1956).

SMITH, R. T. and BRIDGES, R. A.: Immunological unresponsiveness in rabbits produced by neonatal injection of defined antigens. J. exp. Med. 108: 227 250 (1958).

SMITH, S. B.; ISAKOVIĆ, K. and WAKSMAN, B. H.: Role of the thymus in tolerance. II. Transfer of specific unresponsiveness to BSA with thymus grafting. Proc. Soc. exp. Biol., N. Y. 121: 1005–1008 (1966).

SMITHIES, O.: Antibody induction and tolerance. Science 149: 151–156 (1965).

SNELL, G. D.; WINN, H. J.; STIMPFLING, J. H. and PARKER, S. J.: DEPRESSION by antibody of the immune response to homografts and its role in immunological enhancement. J. exp. Med. 112: 293–314 (1960).

SOBEY, W. R. and MAGRATH, J. M.: Acquired immunological unresponsiveness to bovine plasma albumin in mice. Austr. J. biol. Sci. 18: 947–951 (1965).

SOBEY, W. R.; MAGRATH, J. M. and REISNER, A. H.: Genetically controlled specific im-munological unresponsiveness. Immunology, Lond. 11: 511–513 (1966).

SOLOMON, J. B.: Actively acquired transplantation immunity in the chick embryo. Nature, Lond. 198: 1171–1173 (1963).

SOLOMON, J. B. and TUCKER, D. F.: Immunological attack by adult cells in the developing chick embryo: influence of the vascularity of the host spleen and of homograft rejection by the embryo on splenomegaly. J. Embryol. exp. Morph. 11: 119–134 (1963).

SOREM, G. L. and TERRES, G.: The temporal relationship of acquired tolerance and the immune response following injection of bovine serum albumin into neonatal mice. J. Immunol. 90: 217–223 (1963).

SPEISER, P.: Über Antikörperbildung von Säuglingen und Kleinkindern gegen mütter-liches γ_2-Globulin. Ein bisher unbekanntes, dem Erythroblastosemechanismus kon-träres Phänomen mit anscheinend immunogenetisch obligatem Charakter. Wien. med. Wschr. 113: 966–971 (1963).

SPEISER, P. und MICKERTS, D.: Beobachtungen über gehäuftes Auftreten von anti-Gm bei bis zu 2 Jahre alten Kindern nebst Untersuchungen über Antigenverwandtschaft zwischen Gm (a) und Gm (x) mit Pocken-, BCG und Poliomyelitis Antigenen. Blut 10: 425–431 (1964).

STAPLES, P. J.; GERY, I. and WAKSMAN, B. H.: Role of the thymus in tolerance. III. Toler-ance to bovine gamma globulin after direct injection of antigen into the shielded thymus of irradiated rats. J. exp. Med. 124: 127–139 (1966).

STARK, O. K.: Studies on pneumococcal polysaccharide. II. Mechanism involved in pro-duction of 'immunological paralysis' by type I pneumococcal polysaccharide. J. Im-munol. 74: 130–133 (1955).

ŠTARK, O.; KŘEN, V. and FRENZL, B.: Formation of isohaemagglutinins by chicks tolerant to homologous skin grafts. Folia biol., Praha 6: 64–65 (1960).

ŠTARK, O.; KŘEN, V. and FRENZL, B. Dissociation of isohaemagglutinin formation and tolerance of skin grafts in chicks. Nature, Lond. 190: 281–282 (1961 a).

ŠTARK, O.; KŘEN, V. and FRENZL, B.: Dissociation of two types of immunological toler-ance induced in newborn chicks. Transplant. Bull. 28: 472–474 (1961 b).

ŠTARK, O.; KŘEN, V.; FRENZL, B. and BRDIČKA, R.: Attempt to induce a 'graft-versus-host' reaction in grown tolerant chicks and the causes of its failure. Folia biol., Praha 7: 243–251 (1961 c).

Štark, O.; Křen, V.; Frenzl, B. and Brdička, R.: Split tolerance in chicks; in Mechanisms of Immunological Tolerance, p. 123 (Publ. House Czech. Acad. Sci., Prague 1962).

Steinberg, A. G. and Wilson, J. A.: Hereditary globulin factors and immune tolerance in man. Science *140:* 303–304 (1963).

Šterzl, J.: The demonstration and biological properties of the tissue precursor of serum antibodies. Folia biol., Praha *1:* 193–205 (1955).

Šterzl, J.: Immunological tolerance as the result of terminal differentiation of immunologically competent cells. Nature, Lond. *209:* 416–417 (1966).

Šterzl, J.; Mandel, L.; Miler, I. and Říha, I.: Development of immune reactions in the absence or presence of an antigenic stimulus; in: Molecular and Cellular Basis of Antibody Formation, p. 351 (Publ. House Czech. Acad. Sci., Prague 1965).

Šterzl, J. and Říha, I.: Detection of cells producing 7S antibodies by the plaque technique. Nature, Lond. *208:* 858–859 (1965).

Šterzl, J. and Trnka, Z.: Effect of very large doses of bacterial antigen on antibody production in newborn rabbits. Nature, Lond. *179:* 918–919 (1957).

Stevens, K. M.; Pietryk, H. C. and Cininera, J. L.: Acquired immunological tolerance to a protein antigen in chickens. Brit. J. exp. Path. *39:* 1–7 (1958).

Stone, S. H.: Transfer of allergic encephalomyelitis by lymph node cells in inbred guinea pigs. Science *134:* 619–620 (1961).

Stormont, C.; Weir, W. C. and Lane, L. L.: Erythrocyte mosaicism in a pair of sheep twins. Science *118:* 695–696 (1953).

Streilein, J. W. and Hildreth, E. A.: Tolerance to bovine γ-globulin in adult guinea pigs. J. Immunol. *96:* 1027–1034 (1966).

Sulzberger, M. B.: Zur Frage der experimentellen Salvarsan Überempfindlichkeit. Klin. Wschr. *8:* 253–254 (1929 a).

Sulzberger, M. B.: Hypersensitiveness to neoarphenamine in guinea pigs: experiments in prevention and in desensitization. Arch. Derm. Syph., Berl. *20:* 669–697 (1929 b).

Svoboda, J.: Analysis of acquired tolerance to the Rous sarcoma virus in ducks. I. The effect of intraembryonal and postembryonal injections of fowl blood, lyophilized blood and sheep erythrocytes. Folia biol., Praha *4:* 205–208 (1958).

Svoboda, J.: Basic aspects of the interaction of oncogenic viruses with heterologous cells. Int. Rev. exp. Path. *5:* 25–66 (1966).

Svoboda, J. and Hašek, M.: Influencing the transplantability of the virus of *Rous sarcoma* by immunological approximation in turkey. Folia biol., Praha *2:* 256–284 (1956).

Szenberg, A. and Warner, N. L.: Breakdown of polyvalent tolerance in the chicken by thymic grafts. Nature, Lond. *198:* 1012–1013 (1963).

Tao, T. and Uhr, J. W.: Capacity of pepsin-digested antibody to inhibit antibody formation. Nature, Lond. *212:* 208–209 (1966).

Taylor, R. B.: An effect of thymectomy on recovery from immunological paralysis. Immunology, Lond. *7:* 595–602 (1964).

Tempelis, C. H.; Wolfe, H. R. and Mueller, A.: The production of immunological unresponsiveness by the intravenous injection of bovine serum albumin into the chick embryo. Brit. J. exp. Path. *39:* 323–327 (1958 a).

Tempelis, C. and Wolfe, H. R.: Antibody production in chickens following injections of embryos with bovine serum albumin. Transplant. Bull. *5:* 23–24 (1958 b).

Tempelis, C.; Wolfe, H. R. and Mueller, A. P.: The effect of dosage and time of injection of a soluble antigen on the production of immunological unresponsiveness in chickens. Brit. J. exp. Path. *39:* 328–333 (1958).

TERASAKI, P. I.; CANNON, J. A. and LONGMIRE, W. P.: The specificity of tolerance to homografts in the chickens. J. Immunol. *81:* 246–252 (1958).

TERPLAN, K. L.; WITEBSKY, E.; ROSE, N. R.; PAINE, J. R. and EGAN, R. W.: Experimental thyroiditis in rabbits, guinea pigs and dogs, following immunization with thyroid extracts of their own and of heterologous species. Amer. J. Path. *36:* 213–239 (1960).

TERRES, G. and HUGHES, W. L.: Acquired immune tolerance in mice to crystalline bovine serum albumin. J. Immunol. *83:* 459–467 (1959).

THOMSEN, O.: Untersuchungen über erbliche Blutgruppenantigene bei Hühnern. Heredity *19:* 243–258 (1934).

THORBECKE, G. J.; SISKIND, G. W. and GOLDBERGER,, N.: The induction in mice of sensitization and immunological unresponsiveness by neonatal injection of bovine gamma globulin. J. Immunol. *87:* 147–151 (1961).

TOULLET, F. T. and WAKSMAN, B. H.: Role of the thymus in tolerance. IV. Specific tolerance to homografts in neonatally thymectomized mice grafted with thymus from tolerant donors. J. Immunol. *97:* 686–692 (1966).

TRAUB, E.: A filterable virus recovered from white mice. Science *81:* 298–299 (1935).

TRAUB, E.: The epidemiology of lymphocytic choriomeningitis in white mice. J. exp. Med. *64:* 183–200 (1936 a).

TRAUB, E.: Persistence of lymphocytic choriomeningitis virus in immune animals and its relation to immunity. J. exp. Med. *63:* 847–861 (1936 b).

TRAUB, E.: Factors influencing the persistence of LCM virus in the blood of mice after clinical recovery. J. exp. Med. *68:* 229–250 (1938).

TRAUB, E.: Epidemiology of the lymphocytic choriomeningitis in a mouse stock observed for four years. J. exp. Med. *69:* 801–817 (1939).

TRAUB, E.: Über den Einfluss der latenten Choriomeningitis-Infektion auf die Entstehung der Lymphomatose bei weissen Mäusen. Zbl. Bakt. Parasitkde (I. Abt.) *147:* 16–25 (1941).

TRIPLETT, E. L.: On the mechanism of immunologic self recognition. J. Immunol. *89:* 505–510 (1962).

TUCKER, E. M.: Chimaerism in sheep; in Blood Groups of Animals, p. 415 (Publ. House Czech. Acad. Sci., Prague 1965).

TURK, J. L. and HUMPHREY, J. H.: Immunological unresponsiveness in guinea pigs. II. The effect of unresponsiveness on the development of delayed type hypersensitivity to protein antigens. Immunology, Lond. *4:* 310–317 (1961).

TURK, J. L. and STONE, S. H.: Implication of the cellular changes in lymph nodes during the development and inhibition of delayed type hypersensitivity. In: AMOS and KOPROWSKI's Cell-Bound Antibodies, pp. 51–59 (Wistar Inst. Press, Philadelphia 1963).

UHR, J. W. and ANDERSON, S. G.: The placenta as a homotransplant. Nature, Lond. *194:* 1292–1293 (1962).

UHR, J. W. and BAUMANN, J. B.: Antibody formation. I. Suppression of antibody formation by passively administered antibody. J. exp. Med. *113:* 935–957 (1961).

UPHOFF, D. E.: Alteration of homograft reaction by a-methopterin in lethally irradiated mice treated with homologous marrow. Proc. Soc. exp. Biol., N. Y. *99:* 651–653 (1958a).

UPHOFF, D. E.: Preclusion of secondary phase of irradiation syndrome by inoculation of fetal hematopoietic tissue following lethal total-body x-irradiation. J. nat. Cancer Inst. *20:* 625–632 (1958 b).

VOISIN, G. A.; KINSKY, R. G. and JANSEN, F. K.: Transplantation immunity: localization in mouse serum of antibodies responsible for haemagglutination, cytotoxicity and enhancement. Nature, Lond. *210:* 138–139 (1966).

Vojtíšková, M. and Lengerová, A.: On the possibility that thymus-mediated alloanti-genic stimulation results in tolerance response. Experienty *21:* 661 (1965).

Vojtíšková, M. and Lengerová, A.: Radiation chimeras and the role of thymus in immunological tolerance. Exp. Hematology, *10:* 30–31 (1966).

Vojtíšková, M. and Pokorná, Z.: Prevention of experimental allergic aspermatogenesis in adult mice. Lancet *i:* 644–645 (1964).

Vojtíšková, M. and Poláčková, M.: An experimental model of the epigenetic mechanism of autotolerance using the H-Y antigen in mice. Folia biol., Praha *12:* 137–140 (1966).

Vojtíšková, M.; Chutná, J.; Rychlíková, M. and Pokorná, Z.: On the possible role of immunological tolerance in the prevention of autoimmune aspermatogenesis. Folia biol., Praha *8:* 207–214 (1962).

Vojtíšková, M.; Viklický, V.; Jirsáková, A.; Nouza, K. and Pokorná, Z.: Amethopterin treatment of experimental allergic aspermatogenesis in mice and morphological changes of lymphoid organs. Folia biol., Praha *11:* 364–370 (1965).

Volkert, M. and Larsen, J. H.: Studies on immunological tolerance to LCM virus. III. Duration and maximal effect of adoptive immunization of virus carriers. Acta path. microbiol. scand. *60:* 577–587 (1964).

Volkert, M. and Larsen, J. H.: Studies on immunological tolerance to LCM virus. VI. Immunity conferred on tolerant mice by immune serum and by grafts of homologous lymphoid cells. Acta path. microbiol. scand. *63:* 172–180 (1965 a).

Volkert, M. and Larsen, J. H.: Immunological tolerance to viruses. Progr. med. Virol. (Karger) *7:* 160–207 (1965 b).

Ward, H. K.; Walsh, R. J. and Kooptzoff, O.: Rh antigens and immunological tolerance. Nature, Lond. *179:* 1352–1353 (1957).

Weigand, H. and Hotchin, J.: Studies of lymphocytic choriomeningitis in mice. II. A comparison of the immune status of newborn and adult mice surviving inoculation. J. Immunol. *86:* 401–406 (1961).

Weigle, W. O.: The immune response of rabbits tolerant to bovine serum albumin to the injection of other heterologous serum albumins. J. exp. Med. *114:* 111–125 (1961).

Weigle, W. O.: Termination of acquired immunological tolerance to protein antigens following immunization with altered protein antigens. J. exp. Med. *116:* 913–928 (1962).

Weigle, W. O.: The effect of x-radiation and passive antibody on immunologic tolerance in the rabbit to bovine serum albumin. J. Immunol. *92:* 113–117 (1964 a).

Weigle, W. O.: Studies on the termination of acquired tolerance to serum protein antigens following injection of serologically related antigens. Immunology, Lond. *7:* 239–247 (1964 b).

Weigle, W. O.: The immune response of rabbits tolerant to one protein conjugate following the injection of related protein conjugates. J. Immunol. *94:* 177–183 (1965a).

Weigle, W. O.: The production of thyroiditis and antibody following injection of unaltered thyroglobulin without adjuvant into rabbits previously stimulated with altered thyroglobulin. J. exp. Med. *122:* 1049 (1965 b).

Weigle, W. O.: The suppression of antibody production to serum protein antigens in guinea pig. Int. Arch. Allergy *29:* 254–259 (1966 a).

Weigle, W. O.: The induction of hyporesponsive state of hemocyanin. J. Immunol. *96:* 319–323 (1966 b).

Weigle, W. O. and Dixon, F. J.: The antibody response of lymph node cells transferred to tolerant recipients. J. Immunol. *82:* 516–519 (1959).

WEIGLE, W. O. and FUDENBERG, H. H.: Specificity of immunological tolerance induced in the rabbit to genetic determinants of human γ_6-globulin. Int. Arch. Allergy 29: 28–35 (1966).

WEISS, D. W.: Inhibition of tuberculin skin hypersensitivity in guinea pigs by injection of tuberculin and intact tubercle bacilli during foetal life. J. exp. Med. 108: 83–103 (1958).

WEISS, D. W. and WELLS, A. Q.: Actively acquired tolerance to tuberculoprotein. Nature, Lond. 179: 968–969 (1957).

WICHER, K. and ROGALOWA, D.: Attempts to induce acquired tolerance to Treponema pallidum in rabbits. Bull. Polish Med. Sci. History 3: 62–66 (1960).

WICHER, K. and WOŹNICZKO-ORŁOWSKA, G.: Are the group isoantibodies titre in children related to the mother's blood groups? (In Polish). Polski Tygodnik lek. 15: (13): 1–7 (1960).

WIGZELL, H.: Antibody synthesis at the cellular level. Antibody-induced suppression of 7S antibody synthesis. J. exp. Med. 124: 953–969 (1966).

WILSON, J. A. and STEINBERG, A. G.: Antibodies to γ-globulin in the serum of children and adults. Transfusion, Philad. 5: 516–524 (1965).

WITEBSKY, E. and ROSE, N. R.: Studies on organ specificity. VII. Production of antibodies to rabbit thyroid by injection of foreign thyroid extracts. J. Immunol. 83: 41–48 (1959).

WOLFE, H. R.; TEMPELIS, C.; MUELLER, A. and REIBEL, S.: Precipitin production in chickens. XVII. The effect of massive injections of bovine serum albumin at hatching on subsequent antibody production. J. Immunol. 79: 147–153 (1957).

WOODRUFF, M. F. A.: Prolonged survival of skin homografts in adult mice following sublethal irradiation, injection of donor strain spleen cells and administration of amethopterin. Nature, Lond. 195: 727–728 (1962).

WOODRUFF, M. F. A.; FOX, M.; BUCTON, K. A. and JACOBS, P. A.: The recognition of human blood chimaeras. Lancet i: 192–194 (1962).

WOODRUFF, M. F. A. and LENNOX, B.: Reciprocal skin grafts in a pair of twins showing blood chimerism. Lancet ii: 476–478 (1959).

YOSHIMURA, M. and CINADER, B.: The effect of tolerance on the specificity of the antibody response: Antibody to oxazolonated albumin of animals tolerant to the protein carrier. J. Immunol. 97: 959–968 (1966).

ZAALBERG, O. B. and VAN DER MEUL, V. A.: Continued immunological tolerance in mice, independent of antigen excess. Transplantation 4: 274–292 (1966).

ZALESKI, M.; ČERNÝ, J. and HRABA, T.: Cytological changes in the regional lymph nodes of rabbits after local administration of human serum albumin. Folia biol. Praha 12: 22–28 (1966).

ZALESKI, M.; RYMASZEWSKA, T.; LOJEK, T. and KURNATOWSKI, W.: Evaluation of the blastic reaction evoked by tissue grafts in regional lymph nodes. Transplantation 2: 207–211 (1964).

ZEISS, I. M.: An analysis of third-party unresponsiveness in immunologically tolerant rats. Immunology, Lond. 11: 597–602 (1966).

ZILBER, L. A.: Suppression of antibody formation against normal and tumour tissues using the method of acquired tolerance; in Mechanisms of Antibody Formation, p. 332 (Publ. House Czech. Acad. Sci., Prague 1962).

Author's address: Dr. T. Hraba, Czechoslovak Academy of Sciences, Institute of Experimental Biology and Genetics, Flemingovo nám. 2, Prague 6 (ČSSR).

APPENDIX

The Technique of Embryonic Parabiosis

The most appropriate time to perform the parabiotic union of the embryos is in chicks and pheasants on the 8–12th day and in ducks and turkeys on the 12–15th day of incubation. At this time the allantochorion has occupied for the greater part the space under the shell, and the period before hatching is long enough for the formation of anastomotic connections joining the two animals and for a sufficiently long-lasting exchange of their blood to be made.

The parabiotic connection is made near the pointed end of the egg so that it does not prevent normal hatching. The appropriate position, i. e., the site of branching of the large chorioallantoid vessels, is determined by transillumination and indicated on the shell surface with a pencil mark. An oval or rhombic window is then cut at the indicated point by means of a portable electric saw with a sterilized blade (Fig. 12). The longer diameter of the hole is 10–12 mm and the shorter about half the longer one. The window is oriented with its longer diameter in parallel to the egg axis. The loosened shell is then carefully removed with the point of the forceps, care being taken that the shell membrane is not damaged. Sterile Ringer's solution or other suitable solution is dropped on to the bared membrane; when the membrane is soaked with the solution, it is pierced with the point of the forceps; care must be taken not to puncture the allantochorion. Through the opening the solution penetrates underneath the shell membrane and separates it from the allantochorion lying beneath it. The shell membrane can then be easily removed with a forceps.

The second egg with an embryo to be joined in parabiosis is prepared in the same way.

Since the contact alone of the allantochorions of two embryos does not lead with sufficient reliability to the formation of vascular anastomoses, a tissue transplant is inserted between the two allantochorionic membranes. As a transplant, the blastoderm from another egg incubated 20–40 h is generally used. Blastoderms from eggs incubated for a shorter time are too fragile and difficult to handle. The egg is left at rest for at least 1 min before the blastoderm is removed so that the blastoderm turns upwards on the yolk. The blastoderm is obtained by breaking the egg and pouring its contents into a Petri dish. When the orientation of the egg is kept, the blastoderm remains on the top of the yolk. The yolk is fixed by holding one chalaza with a forceps. The blastoderm is then cut off with scissors (Fig. 13) and transferred to another dish with Ringer's solution by a spatula. Here the remains

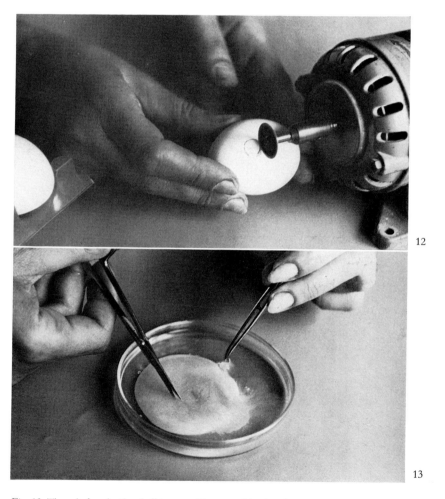

12

13

Fig. 12. The window in the shell is cut with a portable electric saw.
Fig. 13. The blastoderm is cut off from the yolk.

of the yolk are removed and the vitelline membrane is peeled off with a forceps. The cleaned blastoderm is spread over on a spatula and transferred to the allantochorion of one of the prepared eggs (Fig. 14). The egg is held with the pointed end downwards so that the allantochorion would cover the window in the shell and the contents of the egg would bulge slightly. The blastoderm is spread over on the bared allanto-

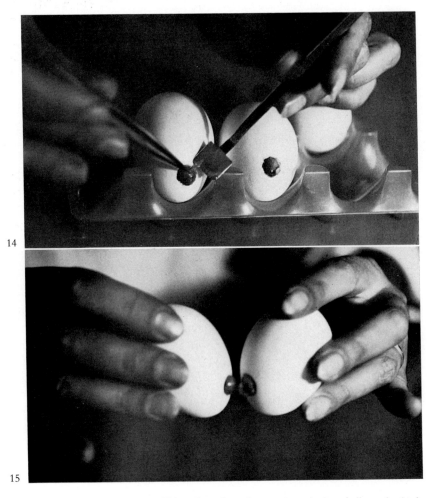

14

15

Fig. 14. Transfer of the isolated blastoderm from the spatula to the bared allantochorionic membrane.
Fig. 15. Two eggs are rolled together with the windows in alignment.

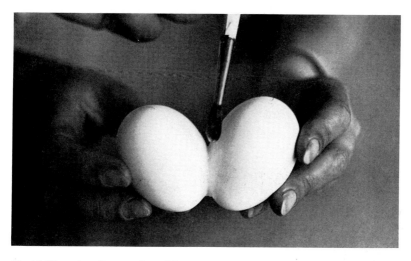

Fig. 16. The point of connection of the two eggs is sealed with melted paraffin wax.

chorion by the aid of a forceps. The graft should not extend beyond the edges of the shell. It could then get in contact with the outer environment and thus an infection could penetrate the egg.

The window in the shell in which the allantochorion is covered with the blastoderm is brought in close contact with the corresponding window of the second egg (Fig. 15). Its allantochorion is also slightly bulging to fit the blastoderm tightly on the allantochorion of the first egg. The eggs are sealed together in this position with paraffin wax (Fig. 16), its temperature being slightly higher than its melting point. Thus the tissues adjacent to the paraffin bridge are not damaged by excessive heat. The paraffin wax is gradually applied in thin layers with a brush until a sufficiently strong bridge is formed capable of preventing undesiderable dislocation. The joined eggs are normally incubated. When the eggs are handled, care must be taken that no displacement at the site of their connection takes place, especially with regard to the fact that paraffin wax grows softer at the temperature of the incubator.

In all cases care must be taken to prevent infection by sealing the shells as tightly as possible and at the same time to avoid covering too much of their surface with the paraffin wax because this would reduce the area of the shell through which the gas is exchanged between the chorioallantoid vessels and the outer environment.

All the operations on the eggs with opened shells must be performed under sterile conditions. The shell at the site of opening and the whole surface of the shell of the egg used for the preparation of the blastoderm are washed with solution of iodine in alcohol.

Hatching of the parabionts generally does not require any further intervention.